A Short Course on

Understanding Your Advanced Cardiovascular Profile Report

By

Kota J. Reddy, M.D.

AUTHOR/WRITER/PUBLISHER: Kota J. Reddy, M.D.
ILLUSTRATOR/WRITER/EDITOR: Joey R. Bangit
EDITOR: Nicolette Groen

FIRST EDITION

DISCLAIMER

The contents and information in this book are for your informational
use only. This program is not intended to be a substitute for
professional medical advice, diagnosis or treatment. Always seek the
advice of your physician, or other qualified health provider with any
questions you may have regarding a medical condition. Never disregard
or delay professional medical advise because of something you have
read in this educational material.

> **"Let food be thy medicine
> and medicine be thy food."**
>
> — HIPPOCRATES (460-370 B.C.)

**Learn to use your food as
your medicine by using your
grocery store as your
pharmacy.**

How?

By reading:

Eat this Lose that!

(SEE APPENDIX FOR MORE INFORMATION)

Congratulations! You have just received an Advanced Cardiovascular Profile test report from Health Diagnostic Laboratory, Inc. This comprehensive panel of advanced tests is a powerful tool for you and your doctor. Using this in-depth menu of tests, your doctor may discover risk indicators in your laboratory results that previous testing never revealed. Since early detection is your first and most promising step to better health, you are on the right track!

This book will guide you in understanding your results, so please take time to read it.

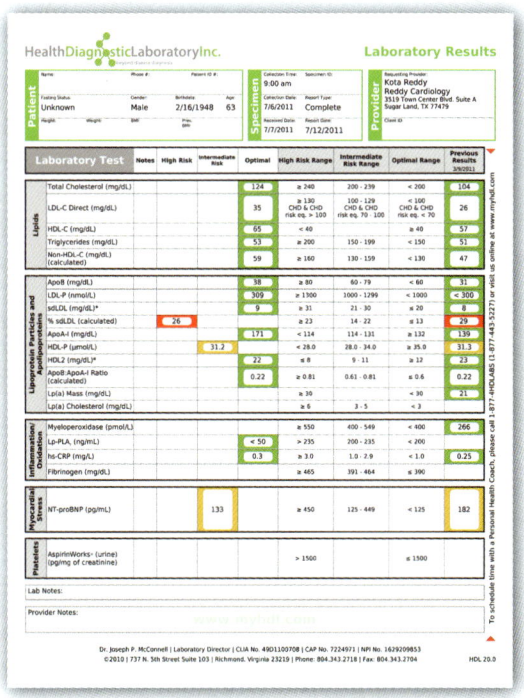

Now, get your Health Diagnostic Laboratory, Inc. report and let's get started!

Contents

introduction

Introduction

Identification, detection, and evaluation of risk factors are an essential part of standard clinical practice in cardiology, and testing for a cholesterol profile of a patient is one of them. Most cardiologists these days only look at your basic cholesterol test to determine your risk of heart disease. Sadly, this is not enough. This is just 10% of the picture. It's like the tip of an iceberg.

Many new emerging cholesterol and non-cholesterol risk factors have been proven to better identify people who are at risk of heart disease. This book will introduce you to the most advanced cardiovascular testing available from Health Diagnostic Laboratory, Inc.

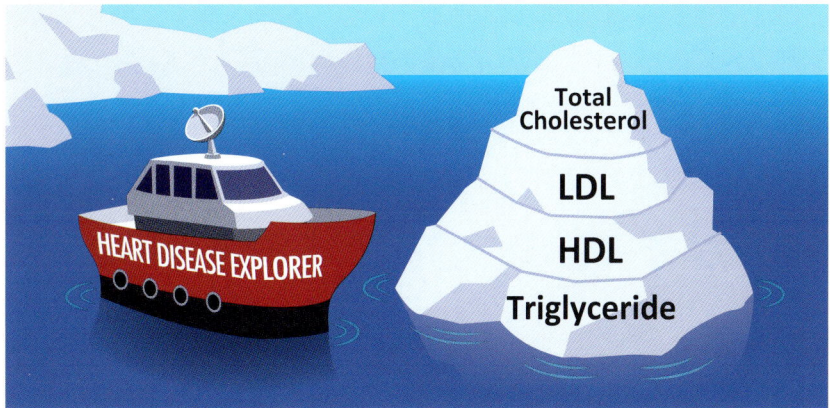

Most cardiologists only look at your basic cholesterol test to determine your risk of heart disease.

NOTE: This test was first introduced in the early '60s.

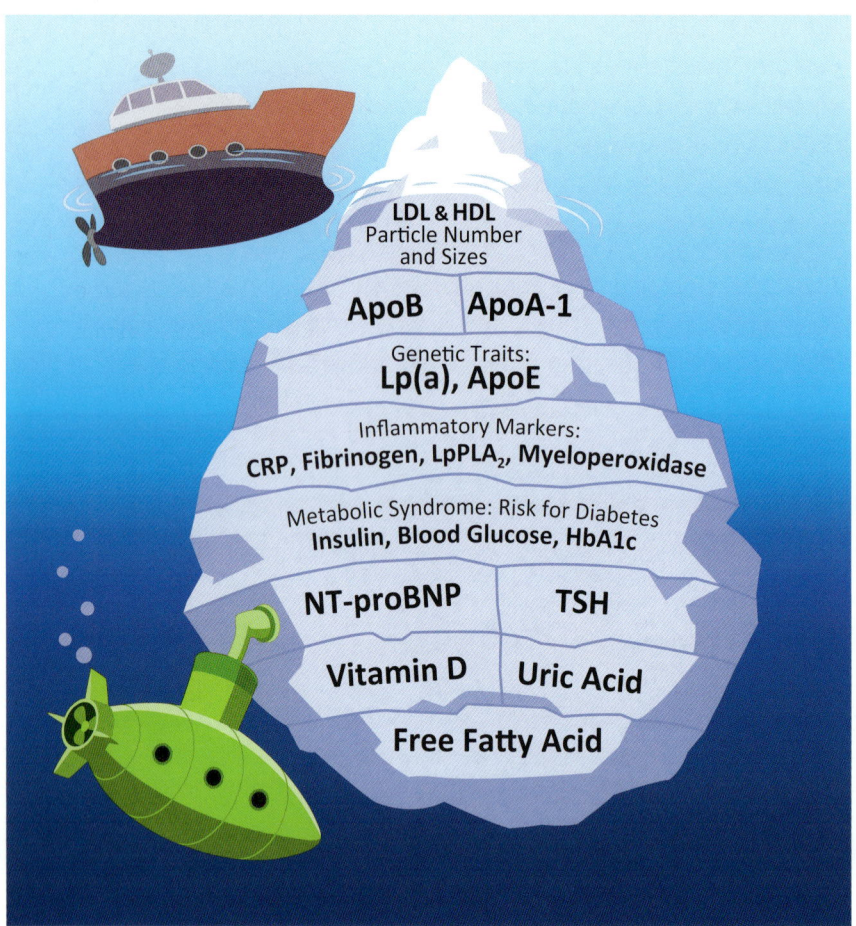

With advanced cardiovascular testing, we'll go deeper so you don't miss the big picture!

HealthDiagnosticLaboratoryInc.
beyond disease diagnosis

Laboratory Results

Name:	Phone #: Patient ID #:
Fasting Status: Unknown	Gender: Male Birthdate: 2/16/1948 Age: 63
BMI:	

Specimen
Collection Time: 9:00 am Specimen ID:
Collection Date: 7/6/2011 Report Type: Complete
Receiv 7/7/

Provider
Requesting Provider:
Kota Reddy
Reddy Cardiology
3519 Town Center Blvd. Suite A
Sugar Land, TX 77479
Client ID:

| **name of test** | **result** | **optimal and risk range** | **previous result** |

Laboratory Test	Notes	High Risk	Intermediate Risk	Optimal	High Risk Range	Intermediate Risk Range	Optimal Range	Previous Results 3/9/2011
Lipids								
Total Cholesterol (mg/dL)				124	≥ 240	200 - 239	< 200	104
LDL-C Direct (mg/dL)				35	≥ 130 CHD & CHD risk eq. > 100	100 - 129 CHD & CHD risk eq. 70 - 100	< 100 CHD & CHD risk eq. < 70	26
HDL-C (mg/dL)				65	< 40		≥ 40	57
Triglycerides (mg/dL)				53	≥ 200	150 - 199	< 150	51
Non-HDL-C (mg/dL) (calculated)				59	≥ 160	130 - 159	< 130	47
Lipoprotein Particles and Apolipoproteins								
ApoB (mg/dL)				38	≥ 80	60 - 79	< 60	31
LDL-P (nmol/L)				309	≥ 1300	1000 - 1299	< 1000	< 300
sdLDL (mg/dL)*				9	≥ 31	21 - 30	≤ 20	8
% sdLDL (calculated)		26			≥ 23	14 - 22	≤ 13	29
ApoA-I (mg/dL)				171	< 114	114 - 131	≥ 132	139
HDL-P (µmol/L)			31.2		< 28.0	28.0 - 34.0	≥ 35.0	31.3
HDL2 (mg/dL)*				22	≤ 8	9 - 11	≥ 12	23
ApoB:ApoA-I Ratio (calculated)				0.22	≥ 0.81	0.61 - 0.81	≤ 0.6	0.22
Lp(a) Mass (mg/dL)					≥ 30		< 30	21
Lp(a) Cholesterol (mg/dL)					≥ 6	3 - 5	< 3	
Inflammation/ Oxidation								
Myeloperoxidase (pmol/L)					≥ 550	400 - 549	< 400	266
Lp-PLA₂ (ng/mL)				< 50	> 235	200 - 235	< 200	
hs-CRP (mg/L)				0.3	≥ 3.0	1.0 - 2.9	< 1.0	0.25
Fibrinogen (mg/dL)					≥ 465	391 - 464	≤ 390	
Myocardial Stress								
NT-proBNP (pg/mL)			133		≥ 450	125 - 449	< 125	182
Platelets								
AspirinWorks® (urine) (pg/mg of creatinine)					> 1500		≤ 1500	

Lab Notes:

Provider Notes:

Dr. Joseph P. McConnell | Laboratory Director | CLIA No. 49D1100708 | CAP No. 7224971 | NPI No. 1629209853
©2010 | 737 N. 5th Street Suite 103 | Richmond, Virginia 23219 | Phone: 804.343.2718 | Fax: 804.343.2704   HDL 20.0

To schedule time with a Personal Health Coach, please call 1-877-4HDLABS (1-877-443-5227) or visit us online

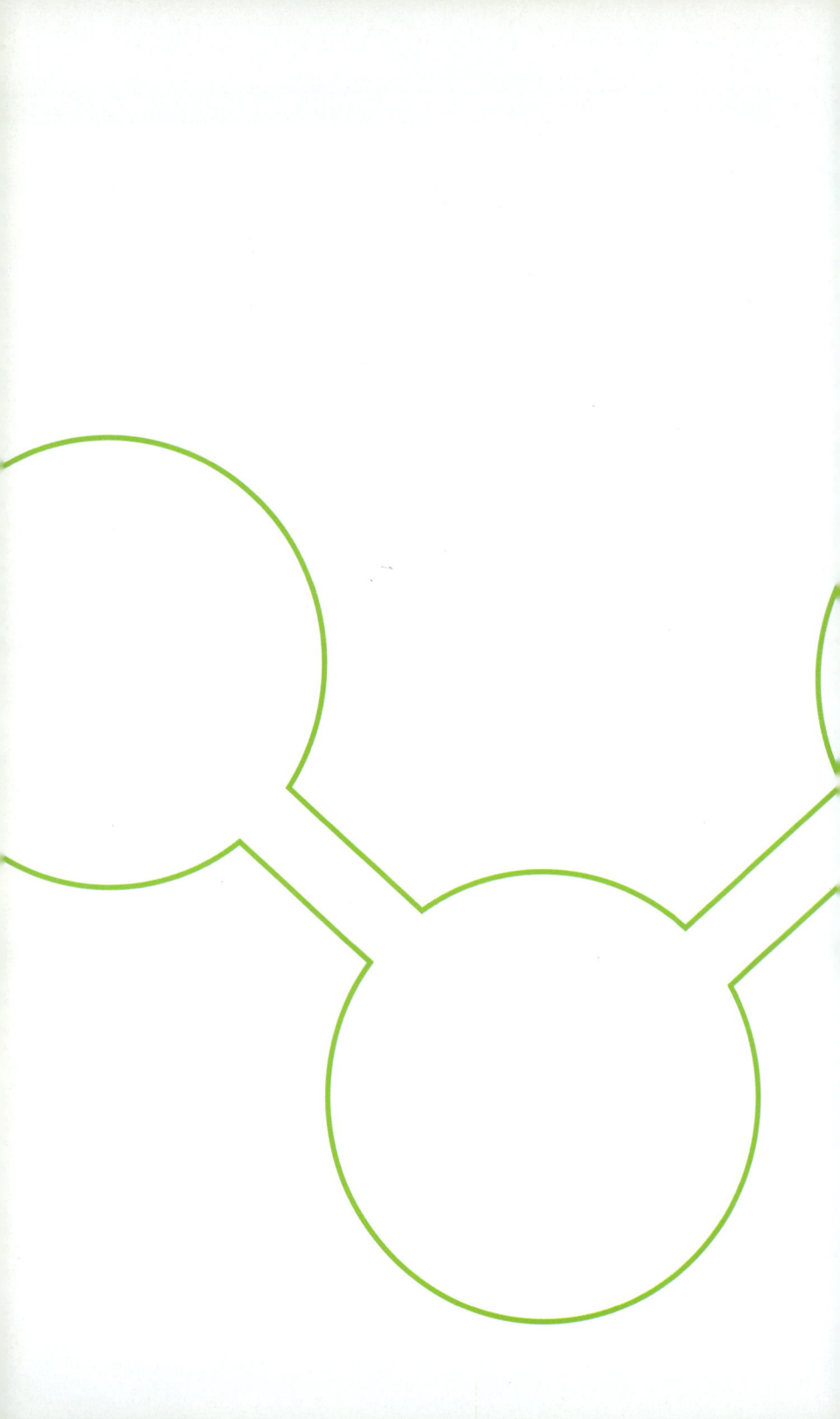

1

lipids

The first test we look for is Total Cholesterol.

Laboratory Test	Notes	High Risk	Intermediate Risk	Optimal	High Risk Range	Intermediate Risk Range	Optimal Range	Previous Results
Total Cholesterol (mg/dL)		262			≥ 240	200 - 239	< 200	
LDL-C Direct (mg/dL)		140			≥ 130 CHD & CHD risk eq. > 100	100 - 129 CHD & CHD risk eq. 70 - 100	< 100 CHD & CHD risk eq. < 70	
HDL-C (mg/dL)				59	< 40		≥ 40	
Triglycerides (mg/dL)				133	≥ 200	150 - 199	< 150	
Non-HDL-C (mg/dL) (calculated)		203			≥ 160	130 - 159	< 130	

What is Total Cholesterol?

Total cholesterol represents the total amount of cholesterol circulating in your blood at the time of the test. It is the summation of your bad cholesterol (LDL-C, low density lipoprotein cholesterol), good cholesterol (HDL-C, high density lipoprotein cholesterol), and ugly cholesterol (triglycerides) divided by 5.

LDL-C + HDL-C + (Triglycerides ÷ 5) = Total Cholesterol

A high cholesterol level in the blood is a major risk factor for heart and blood vessel diseases.

What causes your Total Cholesterol to go up?

The total cholesterol number goes up when the bad cholesterol or good cholesterol go up. The most common cause for elevation in total cholesterol is the combination of sugar, starch, and saturated fat (the bad fat) in the diet, which increases the bad cholesterol.

Laboratory Test	Notes	High Risk	Intermediate Risk	Optimal	High Risk Range	Intermediate Risk Range	Optimal Range	Previous Results
Total Cholesterol (mg/dL)		262			≥ 240	200 - 239	< 200	
LDL-C Direct (mg/dL)		140			≥ 130 CHD & CHD	100 - 129 CHD & CHD	< 100 CHD & CHD	

Your goal should be LESS THAN 150.

LDL cholesterol is also called the **"bad cholesterol."**

Laboratory Test	Notes	High Risk	Intermediate Risk	Optimal	High Risk Range	Intermediate Risk Range	Optimal Range	Previous Results
Total Cholesterol (mg/dL)		262			≥ 240	200 - 239	< 200	
LDL-C Direct (mg/dL)		140			≥ 130 CHD & CHD risk eq. > 100	100 - 129 CHD & CHD risk eq. 70 - 100	< 100 CHD & CHD risk eq. < 70	
HDL-C (mg/dL)				59	< 40		≥ 40	
Triglycerides (mg/dL)				133	≥ 200	150 - 199	< 150	
Non-HDL-C (mg/dL) (calculated)		203			≥ 160	130 - 159	< 130	

"L" for "Lousy." LDLs make a big mess inside the artery by leaving their trash (LDL cholesterol) to pile up and form plaque. A high LDL cholesterol level increases your chances of developing heart disease and stroke.

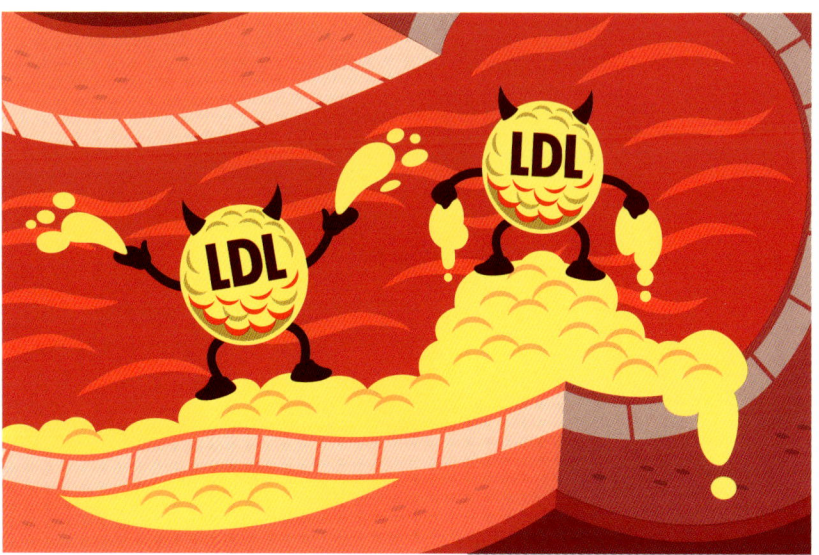

The optimum level for LDL cholesterol is <100mg/dL. But your goal should be less than 70mg/dL to prevent and reverse heart disease.

Your goal should be **LESS THAN 70.**

What causes your LDL Cholesterol to go up?

Diet that includes mostly saturated fat is the most common cause for elevation in LDL cholesterol. Also, eating sugar and starch can increase your small dense LDL cholesterol.

Taking medication like statins (e.g., Lipitor®, Zocor®, Crestor®, etc.) can help you lower this level.

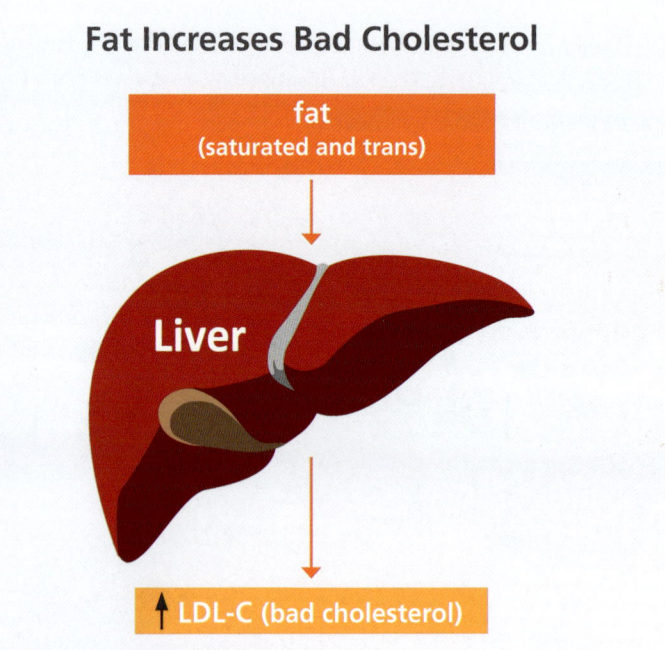

Fat Increases Bad Cholesterol

* Sugar and starch increase small dense LDL cholesterol.

NOTE: 80% of the cholesterol in your diet is not absorbed and therefore will not increase your LDL cholesterol level. It is the saturated fat in your diet that increases the LDL cholesterol level.

HDL Cholesterol is also called the "good cholesterol."

Laboratory Test	Notes	High Risk	Intermediate Risk	Optimal	High Risk Range	Intermediate Risk Range	Optimal Range	Previous Results
Total Cholesterol (mg/dL)		262			≥ 240	200 - 239	< 200	
LDL-C Direct (mg/dL)		140			≥ 130 CHD & CHD risk eq. > 100	100 - 129 CHD & CHD risk eq. 70 - 100	< 100 CHD & CHD risk eq. < 70	
HDL-C (mg/dL)				59	< 40		≥ 40	
Triglycerides (mg/dL)				133	≥ 200	150 - 199	< 150	
Non-HDL-C (mg/dL) (calculated)		203			≥ 160	130 - 159	< 130	

"H" for "Happy." The higher the HDL-C, the longer you live. The lower the HDL-C, the faster you develop heart disease or strokes. The average range of HDL-C is anywhere from 37 to 79mg/dL.

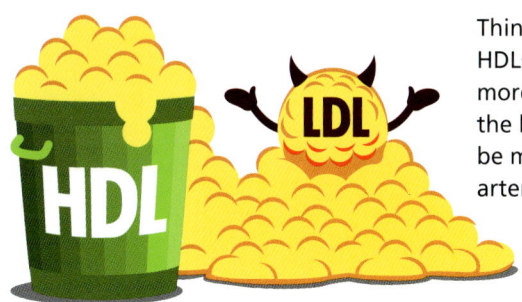

Think of LDL-C as garbage and HDLs as garbage cans. The more garbage cans there are, the better, because there will be more HDLs cleaning the arteries.

What decreases your HDL Cholesterol?

The combination of sugar and starch in your diet destroys HDL cholesterol.

What raises your HDL Cholesterol?

- Diet low in sugar, starch, and trans fat
- Exercise
- Medication in the form of niacin

Your goal should be MORE THAN 60.

Triglycerides are fats in the blood.

Laboratory Test	Notes	High Risk	Intermediate Risk	Optimal	High Risk Range	Intermediate Risk Range	Optimal Range	Previous Results
Total Cholesterol (mg/dL)		262			≥ 240	200 - 239	< 200	
LDL-C Direct (mg/dL)		140			≥ 130 CHD & CHD risk eq. > 100	100 - 129 CHD & CHD risk eq. 70 - 100	< 100 CHD & CHD risk eq. < 70	
HDL-C (mg/dL)				59	< 40		≥ 40	
Triglycerides (mg/dL)				133	≥ 200	150 - 199	< 150	
Non-HDL-C (mg/dL) (calculated)		203			≥ 160	130 - 159	< 130	

What increases your Triglycerides?

Your triglycerides go up if you eat a diet rich in sugar, starch, or saturated fat. The range of triglycerides is anywhere from 72 to 262. Preferably, the triglyceride level should be less than 150, ideally it should be less than 60.

Triglycerides change from meal to meal. If you eat rice, bread, pasta, fruits, chips, cookies, or alcohol the night before, your triglycerides will increase to about 300 to 400 the next day. On the other hand, if your diet is low or devoid of sugar and starch, your triglycerides the next day will be in the 40s or 60s.

What happens when your Triglyceride level is high?

There is an inverse relationship between triglycerides and HDL-C, the good cholesterol. The higher the triglycerides, the lower the good cholesterol. Also, every time the triglycerides go up, the bad cholesterol particles tend to be smaller in size. This is dangerous because high levels of small LDL particles are associated with increasing plaque formation in the arteries.

Your goal should be LESS THAN 60.

Non-HDL Cholesterol tells you how much bad cholesterol is circulating in your blood.

This includes your LDL cholesterol but also your VLDL (very low-density lipoprotein), IDL (intermediate density lipoprotein), and lipoprotein(a) cholesterol levels as well. These are all "bad" cholesterols because they

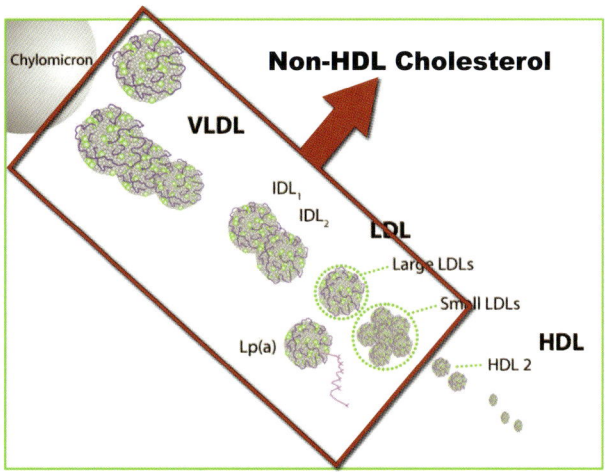

can form plaque and clog the arteries. Non-HDL cholesterol is now considered to be a stronger predictor of cardiovascular disease than LDL cholesterol or triglycerides.

Non-HDL cholesterol is calculated by subtracting HDL-C (good cholesterol) from total cholesterol.

Total Cholesterol – HDL-C = Non-HDL Cholesterol

How do you decrease your Non-HDL Cholesterol?

You can decrease this level by eliminating sugar and starch from your diet.

Your goal should be LESS THAN 130.
(Preferably less than 100)

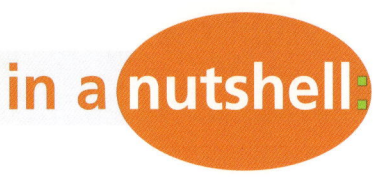

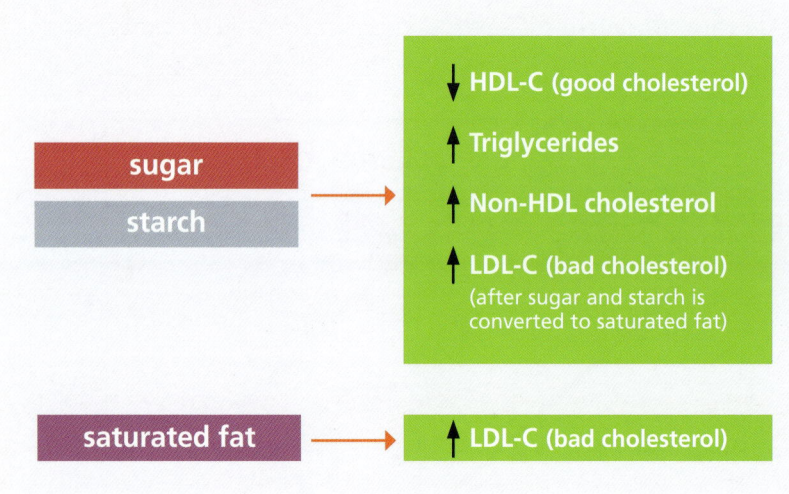

RECOMMENDATION: Learn more about sugar, starch, and saturated fat and how to avoid them by reading the book *Eat This, Lose That* by Kota J. Reddy, M.D. (available at www.reddybread.com).

2

particle sizes and apolipoproteins

LDL-P measures the number of LDL particles in your blood.

Laboratory Test	Notes	High Risk	Intermediate Risk	Optimal	High Risk Range	Intermediate Risk Range	Optimal Range	Previous Results
ApoB (mg/dL)		132			≥ 80	60 - 79	< 60	
LDL-P (nmol/L)		2500			≥ 1300	1000 - 1299	< 1000	
sdLDL (mg/dL)*		38			≥ 31	21 - 30	≤ 20	
% sdLDL (calculated)		27			≥ 23	14 - 22	≤ 13	
ApoA-I (mg/dL)				166	< 130	130 - 150	≥ 151	
HDL-P (μmol/L)				35.5	< 28.0	28.0 - 34.0	≥ 35.0	
HDL2 (mg/dL)*			14		≤ 12	13 - 16	≥ 17	
ApoB:ApoA-I Ratio (calculated)			0.8		≥ 0.81	0.61 - 0.81	≤ 0.6	
Lp(a) Mass (mg/dL)		107			≥ 30		< 30	
Lp(a) Cholesterol (mg/dL)		28						

Lipoprotein Particles and Apolipoproteins

The LDL particle is not the same as LDL cholesterol. Since cholesterol and triglycerides are fatty oils that by themselves cannot dissolve in blood (oil and water do not mix), they need vehicles to travel in the bloodstream. That is why LDL cholesterol and triglycerides are packed into particles.

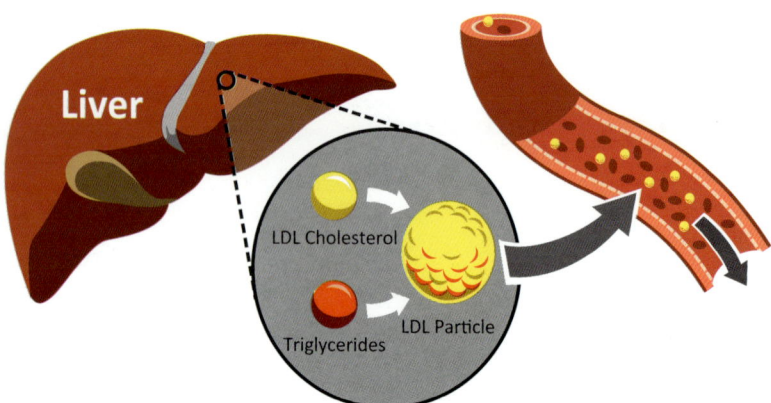

Another way to understand this concept is through this analogy:

Imagine the cars on a freeway. The cars are the LDL particles while the passengers are the LDL cholesterol and triglycerides. The cars will take the passengers where they need to go. Similarly, the LDL particles transport the LDL cholesterol along with triglycerides to every organ in the body, including the arteries.

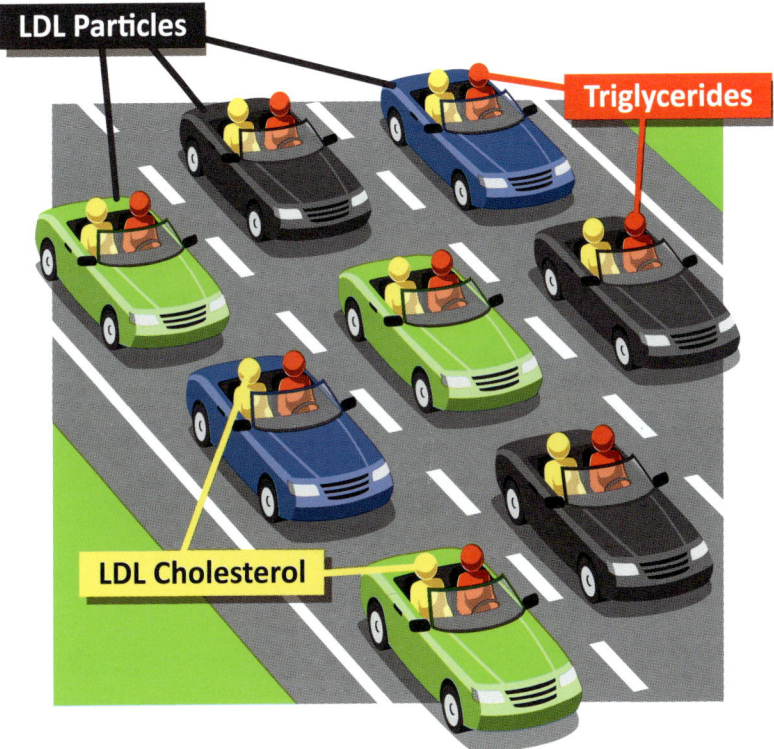

When you measure your cholesterol levels in a regular laboratory, you only measure the number of passengers. This is not enough. You need to measure the number of cars too because they are the drivers of the disease. They deliver the bad cholesterol inside the walls of the artery to form plaque. The more particle numbers you have, the greater your risk for heart disease.

Two patients with the same LDL cholesterol may have different level of risk because they have different LDL particle numbers. Patient A is at low risk for heart disease because he has few LDL particles while Patient B is at high risk because he has many LDL particles.

Let us follow the analogy above:

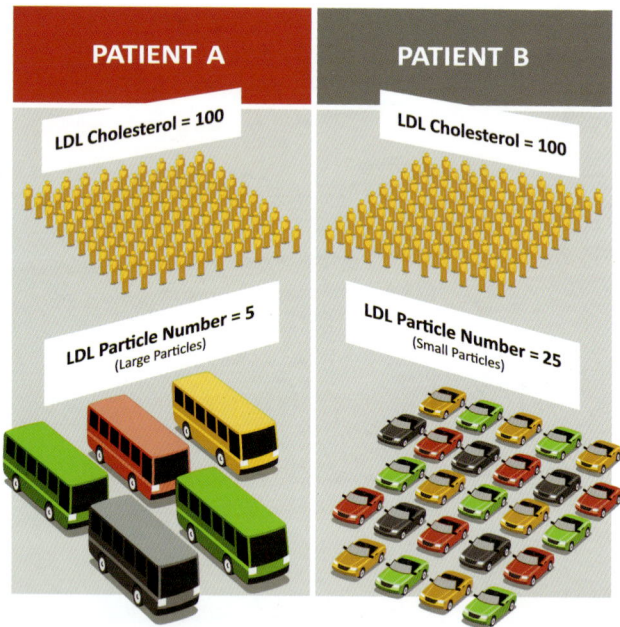

Both patients have 100 passengers. Patient A has 5 buses to carry all his passengers while Patient B has 25 cars to carry his passengers. Patient B is at greater risk for heart disease even though they have the same cholesterol level because he has more vehicles to drive the LDL cholesterol into the artery wall.

As you can see, LDL particles differ in size. Studies have shown that although the small LDL particles contain less LDL cholesterol, they are actually more likely to damage your artery walls than the larger LDL particles.

Your goal should be LESS THAN 1,000.
(Preferably less than 700)

The more LDL particles you have over a period of time, the greater the plaque buildup. If you maintain your LDL-P at less than 700, you are very unlikely to form plaque.

LDL-P and Plaque Buildup

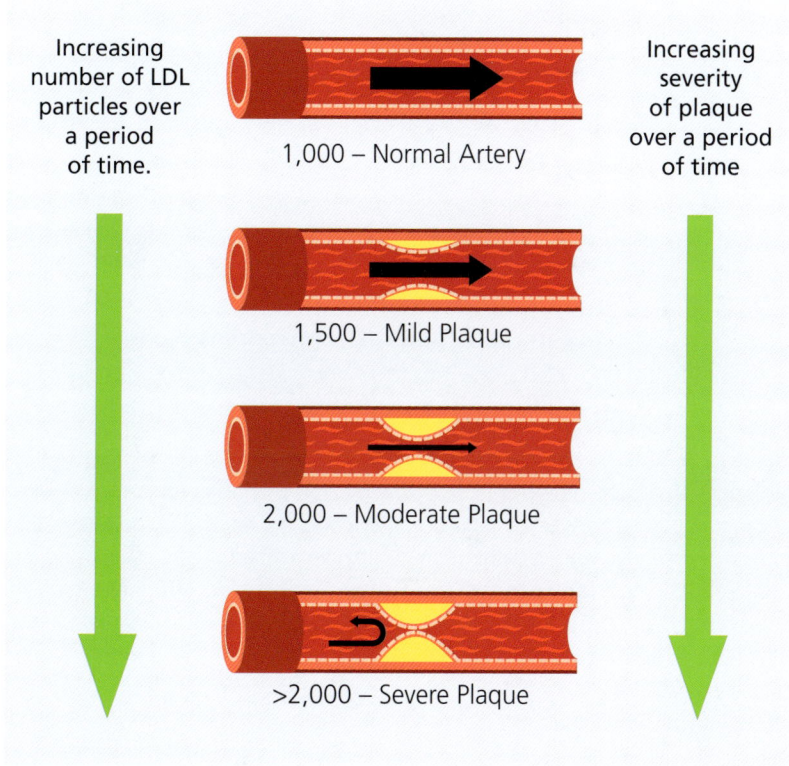

Increasing number of LDL particles over a period of time.

Increasing severity of plaque over a period of time

1,000 – Normal Artery

1,500 – Mild Plaque

2,000 – Moderate Plaque

>2,000 – Severe Plaque

How do you decrease your LDL-P number?

The best way to decrease your LDL-P number other than medication is to eliminate sugar, starch, and saturated fat from your diet (more importantly sugar and starch!).

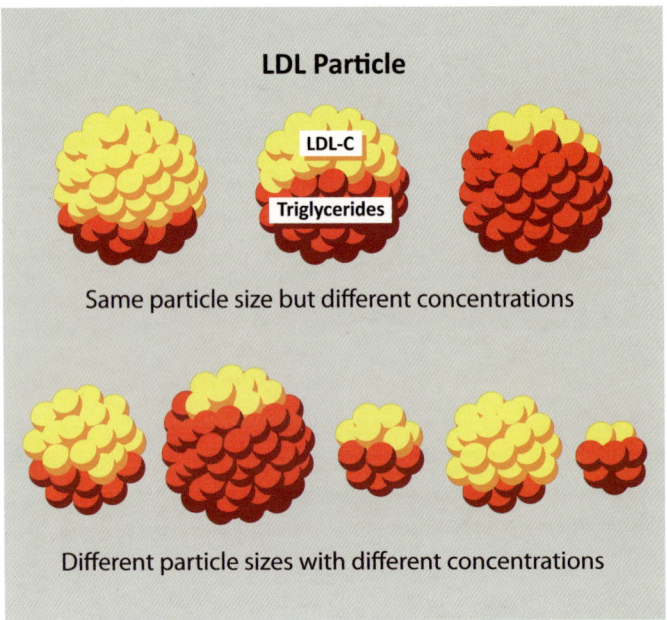

LDL Particle

LDL-C

Triglycerides

Same particle size but different concentrations

Different particle sizes with different concentrations

NOTE: The LDL particles contain different concentrations of LDL cholesterol and triglycerides. The body does not dictate how much LDL cholesterol or triglycerides there should be in a particle. One particle may contain a lot of LDL cholesterol and very few triglycerides while another may contain very little LDL cholesterol and a lot of triglycerides. There is no rule that LDL-P should only contain LDL cholesterol. The point is, even if you have a normal level of LDL cholesterol, your LDL-P number can still be high if your triglyceride level is high. And usually, most of these particles will be small in size.

sdLDL measures the amount of small dense LDL cholesterol present in the body while %sdLDL gives you this value as a percentage of your total cholesterol.

Laboratory Test	Notes	High Risk	Intermediate Risk	Optimal	High Risk Range	Intermediate Risk Range	Optimal Range	Previous Results
ApoB (mg/dL)		132			≥ 80	60 - 79	< 60	
sdLDL (mg/dL)*		38			≥ 1300	1000 - 1299	< 1000	
% sdLDL (calculated)		27			≥ 31	21 - 30	≤ 20	
% sdLDL (calculated)		27			≥ 23	14 - 22	≤ 13	
ApoA-I (mg/dL)				166	< 130	130 - 150	≥ 151	
HDL-P (μmol/L)				35.5	< 28.0	28.0 - 34.0	≥ 35.0	
HDL2 (mg/dL)*			14		≤ 12	13 - 16	≥ 17	
ApoB:ApoA-I Ratio (calculated)				0.8	≥ 0.81	0.61 - 0.81	≤ 0.6	
Lp(a) Mass (mg/dL)		107			≥ 30		< 30	
Lp(a) Cholesterol (mg/dL)		28						

Lipoprotein Particles & Apolipoproteins

Imagine the large LDL particles as rocks and the small dense LDL particles as fine salt and sand. If you were to hold them in your hand, which do you think would go through your fingers? Sand and salt will filter through your hand and fall to the ground.

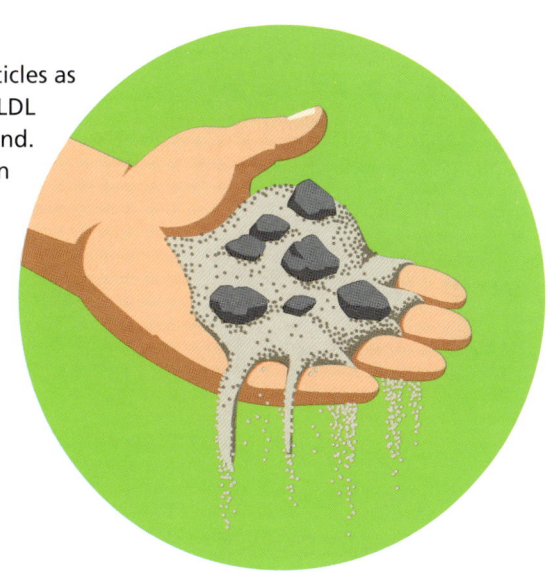

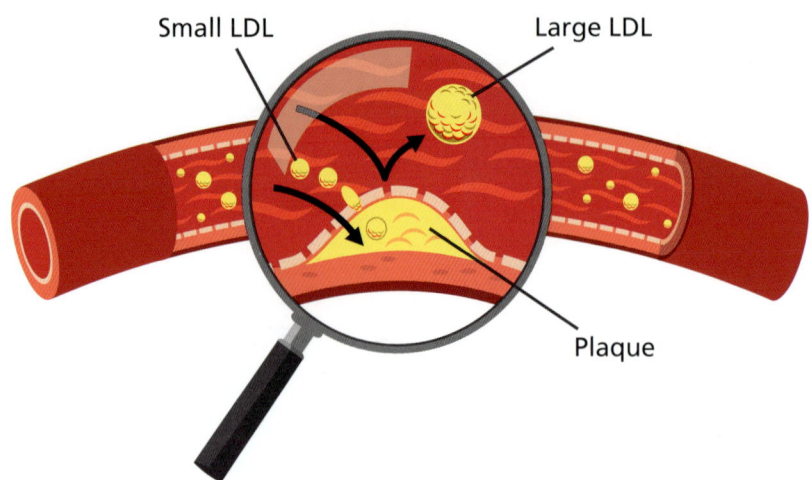

Similarly, if the artery is loaded with different sizes of LDL particles, which particle would you think will pass through the artery wall and form plaque? The small dense particles will easily pass through the cells of the wall because of their small size. Increased number of small dense LDL is dangerous because it makes plaque form much faster.

What makes your LDL particle small in size?

The combination of sugar and starch in your diet tends to make the bad cholesterol particles smaller in size. A high sdLDL or % sdLDL number tells you that you have too many small dense LDL particles.

Your goal should be:

sdLDL	Less than 20mg/dL (preferably less than 15mg/dL)
%sdLDL	Less than 13% (preferably less than 10%)

The lower the better!

HDL-P measures the number of HDL particles in your blood.

Laboratory Test	Notes	High Risk	Intermediate Risk	Optimal	High Risk Range	Intermediate Risk Range	Optimal Range	Previous Results
ApoB (mg/dL)		132			≥ 80	60 - 79	< 60	
LDL-P (nmol/L)		2500			≥ 1300	1000 - 1299	< 1000	
sdLDL (mg/dL)*		38			≥ 31	21 - 30	≤ 20	
% sdLDL (calculated)		27			≥ 23	14 - 22	≤ 13	
ApoA-I (mg/dL)				166	< 130	130 - 150	≥ 151	
HDL-P (µmol/L)				35.5	< 28.0	28.0 - 34.0	≥ 35.0	
HDL2 (mg/dL)*			14		≤ 12	13 - 16	≥ 17	
ApoB:ApoA-I Ratio (calculated)			0.8		≥ 0.81	0.61 - 0.81	≤ 0.6	
Lp(a) Mass (mg/dL)		107			≥ 30		< 30	
Lp(a) Cholesterol (mg/dL)		28						

Lipoprotein Particles and Apolipoproteins

Like LDL cholesterol, HDL cholesterol is packed in particles so it can be transported in the blood. These particles also come in different sizes.

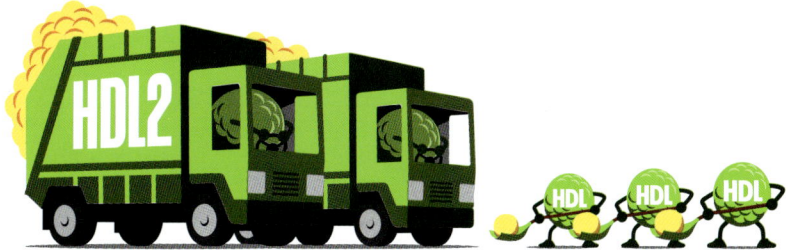

Think of HDL particles as garbage trucks. The more HDL particles you have, the better, because you have more cleaners to clean your artery.

Your HDL-P number increases when you refrain from eating sugar and starch.

Your goal should be **MORE THAN 35.**

HDL2 is the largest and the most effective HDL among its class.

Laboratory Test	Notes	High Risk	Intermediate Risk	Optimal	High Risk Range	Intermediate Risk Range	Optimal Range	Previous Results
ApoB (mg/dL)		132			≥ 80	60 - 79	< 60	
LDL-P (nmol/L)		2500			≥ 1300	1000 - 1299	< 1000	
sdLDL (mg/dL)*		38			≥ 31	21 - 30	≤ 20	
% sdLDL (calculated)		27			≥ 23	14 - 22	≤ 13	
ApoA-I (mg/dL)				166	< 130	130 - 150	≥ 151	
HDL-P (µmol/L)				35.5	< 28.0	28.0 - 34.0	≥ 35.0	
HDL2 (mg/dL)*			14		≤ 12	13 - 16	≥ 17	
ApoB:ApoA-I Ratio (calculated)			0.8		≥ 0.81	0.61 - 0.81	≤ 0.6	
Lp(a) Mass (mg/dL)		107			≥ 30		< 30	
Lp(a) Cholesterol (mg/dL)		28						

Lipoprotein Particles and Apolipoproteins

HDL2 is the workhorse of HDLs. It cleans the arteries more efficiently than smaller HDLs. The more large garbage trucks you have, the cleaner your arteries.

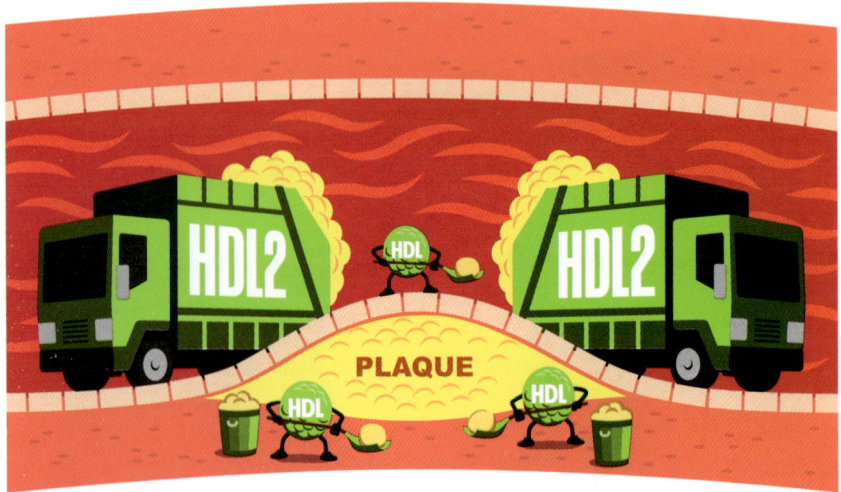

HDL2 takes more cholesterol from plaque and brings it back to the liver for disposal. This is how HDL2 helps accelerate the reversal of heart disease.

Removing Cholesterol From Plaque

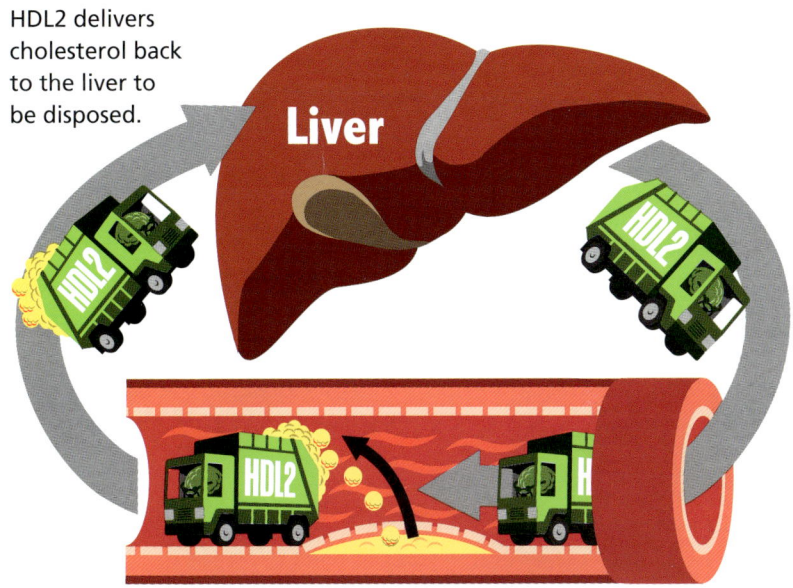

HDL2 delivers cholesterol back to the liver to be disposed.

HDL2 picks up cholesterol from plaque.

What makes your HDL particles small in size?

The combination of sugar and starch in your diet makes your good cholesterol particles small in size, thus decreasing the HDL's ability to remove cholesterol from plaque and clean the artery.

Your goal should be **MORE THAN 17.**

ApoB is a protein cap that each LDL particle wears.

Laboratory Test	Notes	High Risk	Intermediate Risk	Optimal	High Risk Range	Intermediate Risk Range	Optimal Range	Previous Results
ApoB (mg/dL)		132			≥ 80	60 - 79	< 60	
LDL-P (nmol/L)		2500			≥ 1300	1000 - 1299	< 1000	
sdLDL (mg/dL)*		38			≥ 31	21 - 30	≤ 20	
% sdLDL (calculated)		27			≥ 23	14 - 22	≤ 13	
ApoA-I (mg/dL)				166	< 130	130 - 150	≥ 151	
HDL-P (µmol/L)				35.5	< 28.0	28.0 - 34.0	≥ 35.0	
HDL2 (mg/dL)*			14		≤ 12	13 - 16	≥ 17	
ApoB:ApoA-I Ratio (calculated)			0.8		≥ 0.81	0.61 - 0.81	≤ 0.6	
Lp(a) Mass (mg/dL)		107			≥ 30		< 30	
Lp(a) Cholesterol (mg/dL)		28						

It is the "key" that opens the doors of cells and allows the bad cholesterol to come in and form a plaque in your artery.

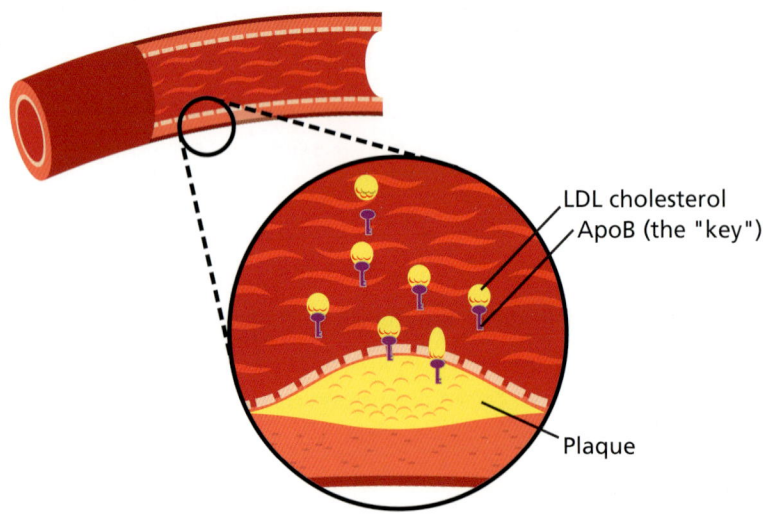

LDL cholesterol
ApoB (the "key")
Plaque

When most of your LDL particles are small in size (due to bad diet), the apoB level tends to be higher. In other words, apoB tells you just how bad your bad cholesterol is. Remember, small LDL particles are very bad because they form plaque faster. Measuring apoB gives you a more precise estimate of your risk for heart disease than measuring LDL-C alone.

high risk

Even though the LDL-C is low, the apoB is high. This means that most of the LDL particles are small, which makes it easier to form plaque.

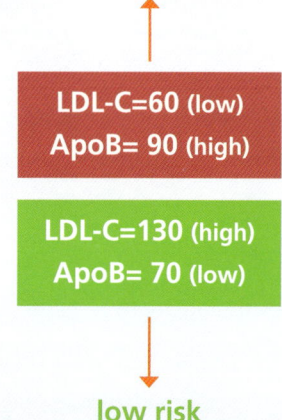

LDL-C=60 (low)
ApoB= 90 (high)

LDL-C=130 (high)
ApoB= 70 (low)

low risk

Even though the LDL-C is high, the apoB is low. This means that most of the LDL particles are big and cannot easily form plaque.

The lower the apoB, the lower the risk for heart disease.

What increases your ApoB?

The combination of sugar and starch in your diet increases your apolipoprotein B level.

Your goal should be LESS THAN 60.

ApoA-1 or Apolipoprotein A-1 is a protein produced in the liver and gut (intestines) that becomes a major component of HDL Particles.

Laboratory Test	Notes	High Risk	Intermediate Risk	Optimal	High Risk Range	Intermediate Risk Range	Optimal Range	Previous Results
ApoB (mg/dL)		132			≥ 80	60 - 79	< 60	
LDL-P (nmol/L)		2500			≥ 1300	1000 - 1299	< 1000	
sdLDL (mg/dL)*		38			≥ 31	21 - 30	≤ 20	
ApoA-1 (mg/dL)				166	≥ 23	14 - 22	≤ 13	
ApoA-1 (mg/dL)				166	< 130	130 - 150	≥ 151	
HDL-P (µmol/L)				35.5	< 28.0	28.0 - 34.0	≥ 35.0	
HDL2 (mg/dL)*			14		< 12			

ApoA-1 gives HDL particles the ability to remove more cholesterol from plaque, thereby cleaning the artery faster. The higher your apoA-1, the better.

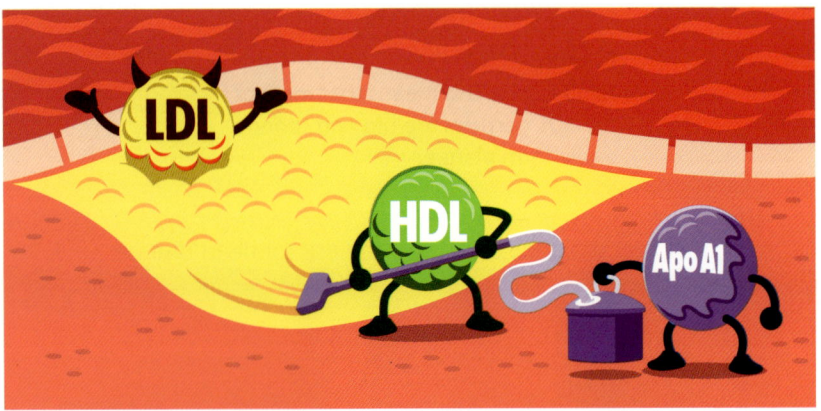

ApoA-1 makes HDL more efficient at cleaning the arteries.

What decreases your ApoA-1?

A low level of apoA-1 is associated with a diet high in sugar and starch and smoking, which leads to early heart and blood vessel diseases.

Your goal should be **MORE THAN 150.**

Lipoprotein(a) or Lp(a) is the worst form of LDL with a very scary protein "corkscrew" attached to it called apoprotein(a).

Laboratory Test	Notes	High Risk	Intermediate Risk	Optimal	High Risk Range	Intermediate Risk Range	Optimal Range	Previous Results
ApoB (mg/dL)		132			≥ 80	60 - 79	< 60	
LDL-P (nmol/L)		2500			≥ 1300	1000 - 1299	< 1000	
sdLDL (mg/dL)*		38			≥ 31	21 - 30	≤ 20	
% sdLDL (calculated)		27			≥ 23	14 - 22	≤ 13	
ApoA-I (mg/dL)				166	< 130	130 - 150	≥ 151	
HDL-P (µmol/L)				35.5	< 28.0	28.0 - 34.0	≥ 35.0	
HDL2 (mg/dL)*			14		≤ 12	13 - 16	≥ 17	
ApoB:ApoA-I Ratio (calculated)			0.8		≥ 0.81	0.61 - 0.81	≤ 0.6	
Lp(a) Mass (mg/dL)		107			≥ 30		< 30	
Lp(a) Cholesterol (mg/dL)		28						

(Left side vertical label: Lipoprotein Particles and Apolipoproteins)

Lp(a) is an inherited trait that can increase heart disease risk.

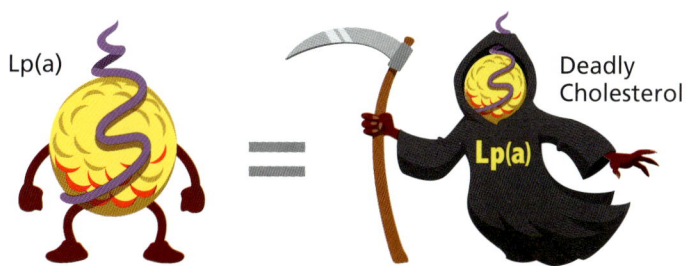

It is so predictive of heart disease that it has been called "the heart attack cholesterol" and "the deadly cholesterol." Researchers at Oxford University in England found that Lp(a) alone can raise your risk of heart attack by as much as 70 percent. It accumulates and promotes the growth of plaque as well as clot formation. Over a prolonged period of time, Lp(a) leads to significant damage to the coronary arteries, thereby making you susceptible to a heart attack.

The level of Lp(a) in your blood is inherited, so it is important that everyone in your family get tested. Furthermore, it does not respond to diet and exercise. One to two grams of niacin daily is the best way to lower its concentration. Hormone replacement therapy with estrogen has also been shown to reduce concentrations of Lp(a) in post-menopausal women.

Lp(a) cholesterol values should not be confused with Lp(a) mass values, although they are highly correlated. Lp(a) cholesterol values will be approximately one tenth that of Lp(a) mass values, but the difference between the measures is not uniform. Lp(a) mass values are considered elevated when >30 mg/dL. Lp(a) cholesterol is increased if > or = 3 mg/dL.

Your goal should be:

Lp(a) mass	Less than 30mg/dL
Lp(a) cholesterol	Less than 3mg/dL

The lower the better!

NOTE: If your Lp(a) is high, but your apoB is very low, you may not be at high risk. Lp(a) is determined by your genes and will remain relatively stable throughout your lifetime, meaning if it is high, it may remain high for as long as you live. Therefore, if you cannot lower your Lp(a), at least keep your apoB as low as possible to lower your risk of heart attack.

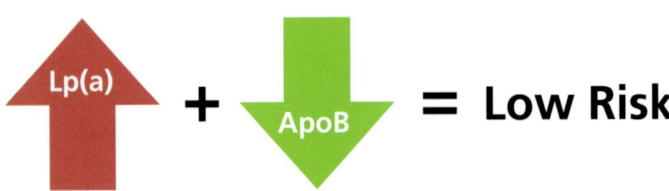

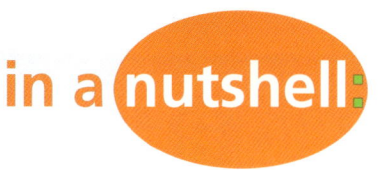

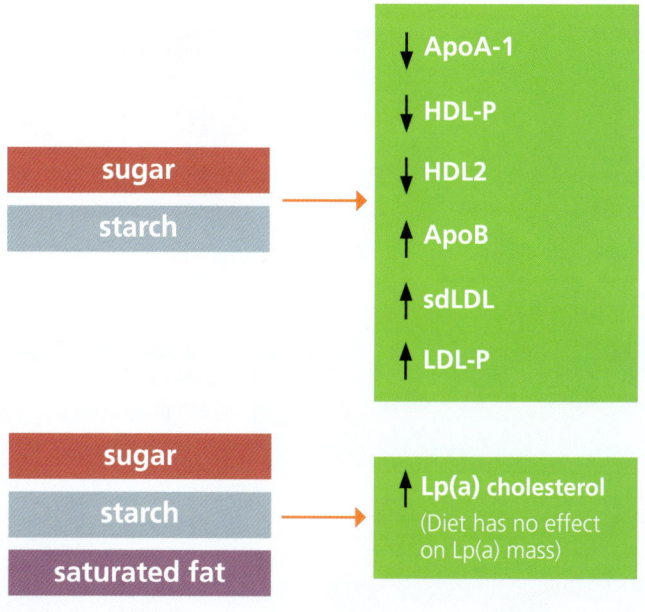

RECOMMENDATION: Learn more about sugar, starch, and saturated fat and how to avoid them by reading the book *Eat This, Lose That* by Kota J. Reddy, M.D. (available at www.reddybread.com).

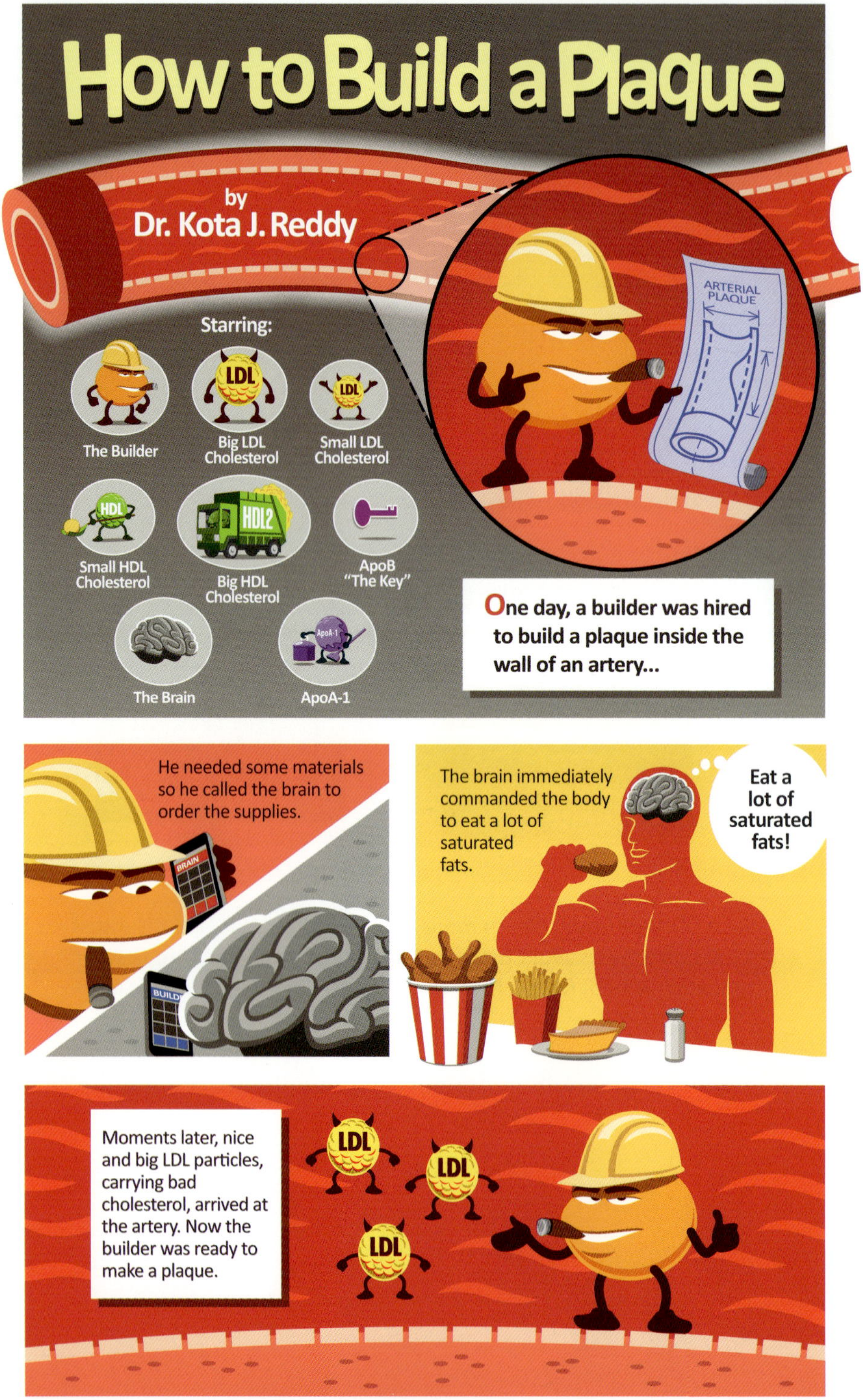

How to Build a Plaque

by
Dr. Kota J. Reddy

Starring:

The Builder

Big LDL Cholesterol

Small LDL Cholesterol

Small HDL Cholesterol

Big HDL Cholesterol

ApoB "The Key"

The Brain

ApoA-1

ARTERIAL PLAQUE

One day, a builder was hired to build a plaque inside the wall of an artery...

He needed some materials so he called the brain to order the supplies.

The brain immediately commanded the body to eat a lot of saturated fats.

Eat a lot of saturated fats!

Moments later, nice and big LDL particles, carrying bad cholesterol, arrived at the artery. Now the builder was ready to make a plaque.

How to Build a Plaque ...

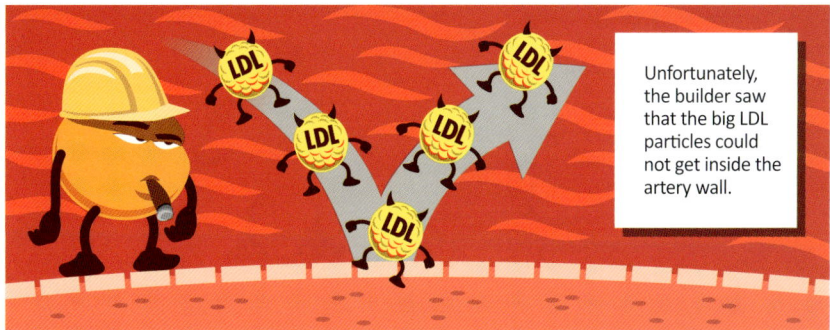

Unfortunately, the builder saw that the big LDL particles could not get inside the artery wall.

He then decided that in order to get the LDL particles inside the wall, it needed to have some sort of...

"key"

So he called the brain again and ordered what he needed...

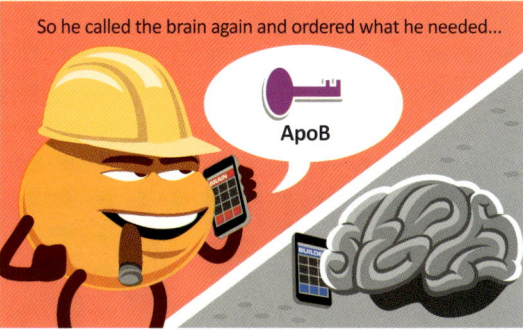

ApoB

The brain immediately commanded the body to eat some sugar and starch.

Eat sugar and starch!

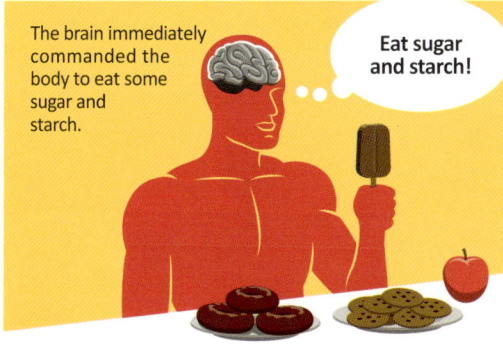

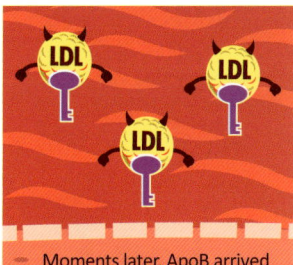

Moments later, ApoB arrived at the artery and attached itself to the LDL particles.

The LDL particles with ApoB could now pass through the wall of the artery. The builder was so happy to see that his plan was working.

How to Build a Plaque ...

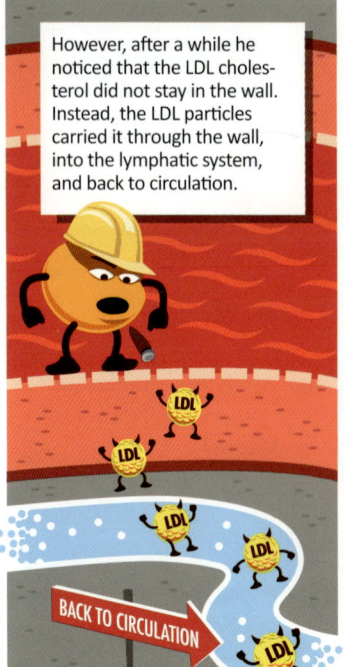

However, after a while he noticed that the LDL cholesterol did not stay in the wall. Instead, the LDL particles carried it through the wall, into the lymphatic system, and back to circulation.

BACK TO CIRCULATION

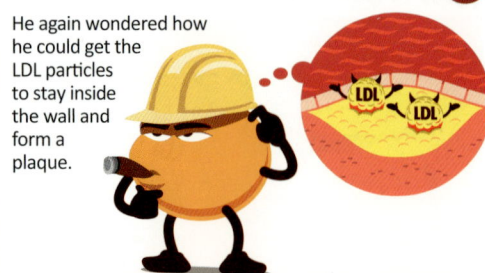

He again wondered how he could get the LDL particles to stay inside the wall and form a plaque.

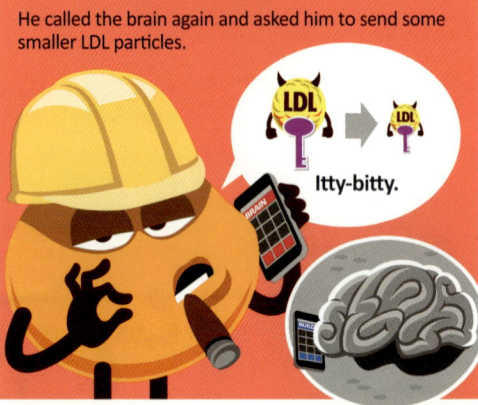

He called the brain again and asked him to send some smaller LDL particles.

Itty-bitty.

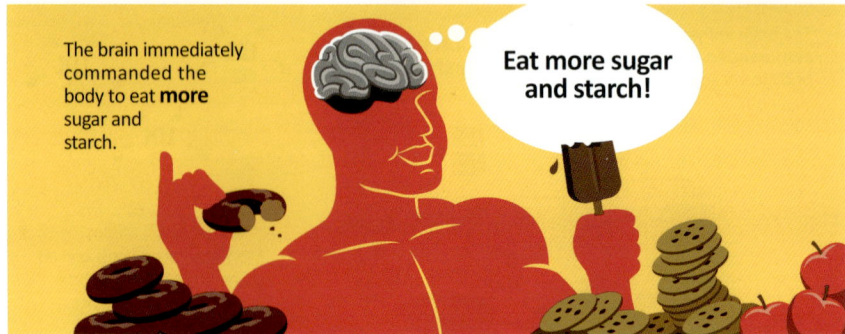

The brain immediately commanded the body to eat **more** sugar and starch.

Eat more sugar and starch!

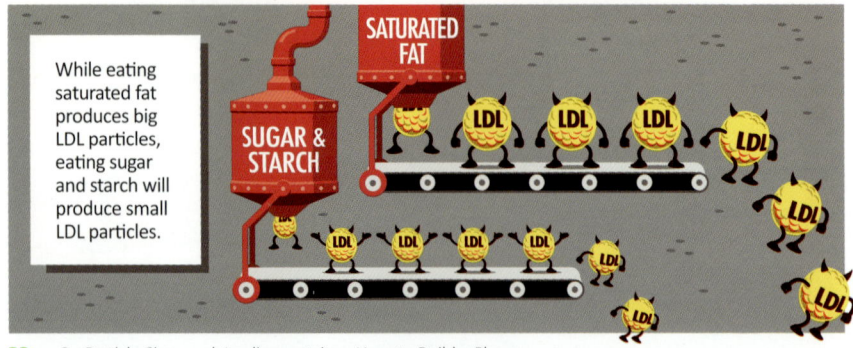

While eating saturated fat produces big LDL particles, eating sugar and starch will produce small LDL particles.

SATURATED FAT

SUGAR & STARCH

How to Build a Plaque

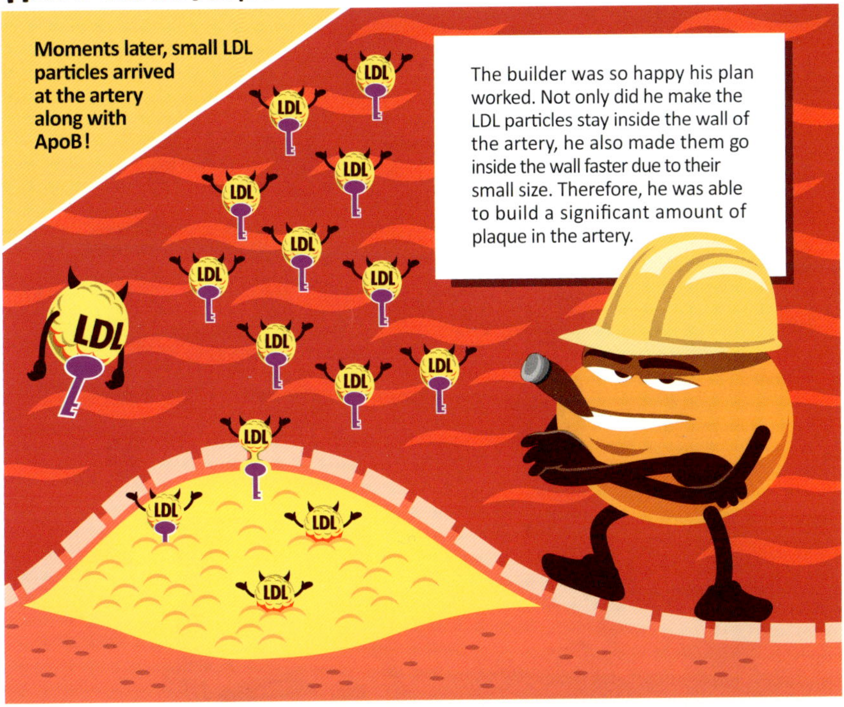

Moments later, small LDL particles arrived at the artery along with ApoB!

The builder was so happy his plan worked. Not only did he make the LDL particles stay inside the wall of the artery, he also made them go inside the wall faster due to their small size. Therefore, he was able to build a significant amount of plaque in the artery.

However, when ApoA-1 detected the plaque in the artery, it immediately alerted the HDL particles to clean the artery.

PLAQUE ALERT!

CLEAN UP! →

ApoA-1

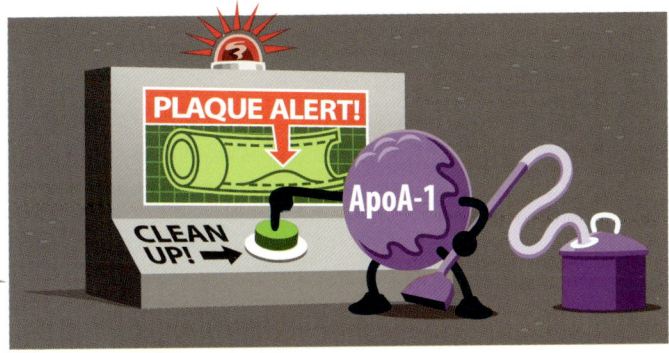

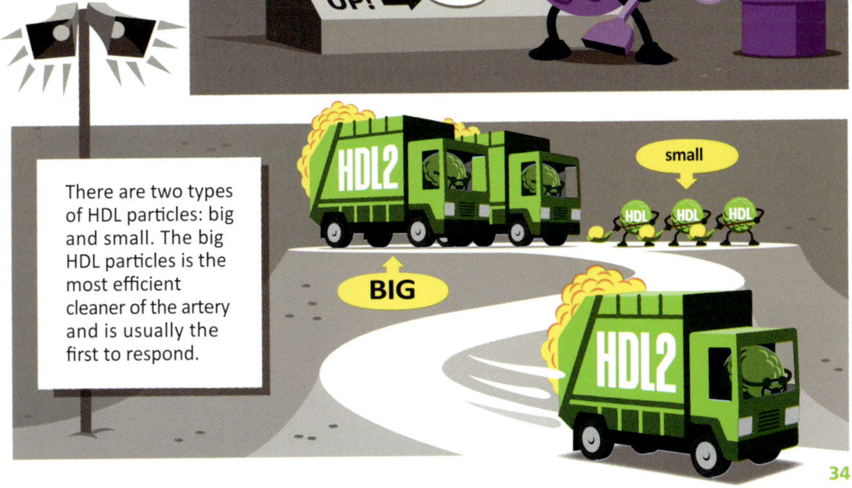

There are two types of HDL particles: big and small. The big HDL particles is the most efficient cleaner of the artery and is usually the first to respond.

HDL2

BIG

small

HDL HDL HDL

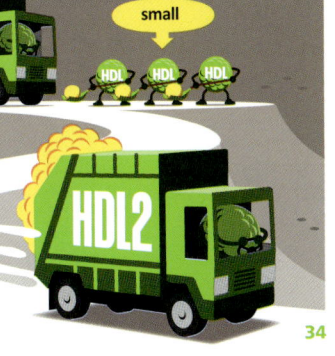

HDL2

How to Build a Plaque

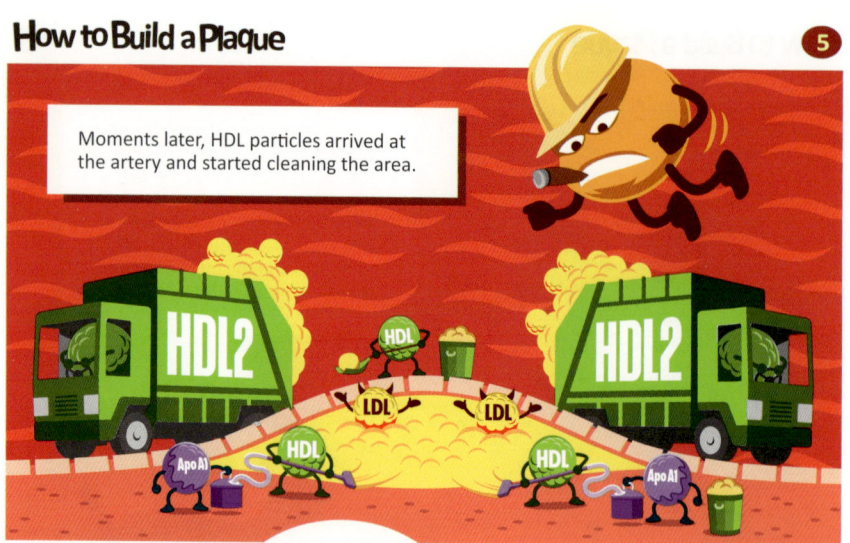

Moments later, HDL particles arrived at the artery and started cleaning the area.

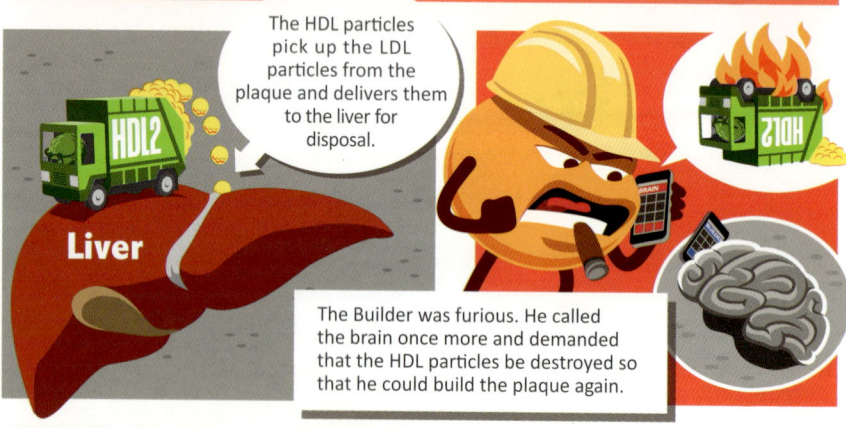

The HDL particles pick up the LDL particles from the plaque and delivers them to the liver for disposal.

Liver

The Builder was furious. He called the brain once more and demanded that the HDL particles be destroyed so that he could build the plaque again.

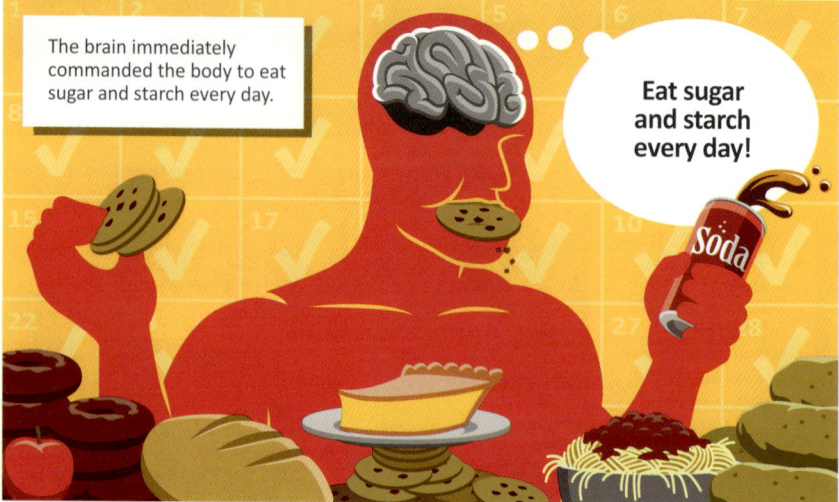

The brain immediately commanded the body to eat sugar and starch every day.

Eat sugar and starch every day!

How to Build a Plaque

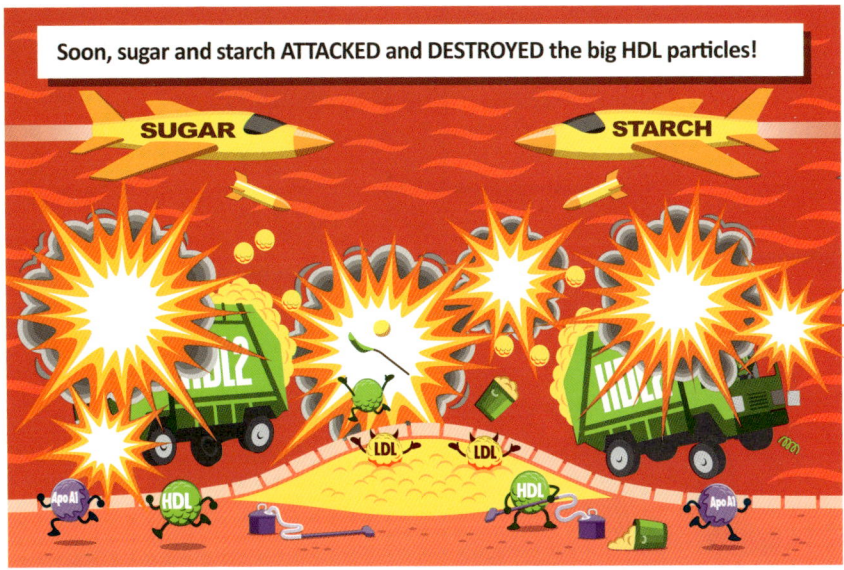

Soon, sugar and starch ATTACKED and DESTROYED the big HDL particles!

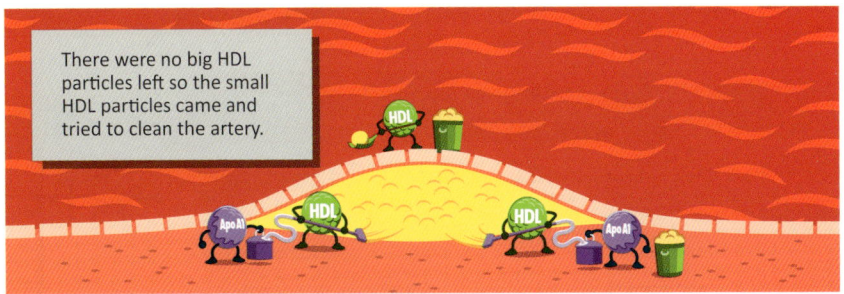

There were no big HDL particles left so the small HDL particles came and tried to clean the artery.

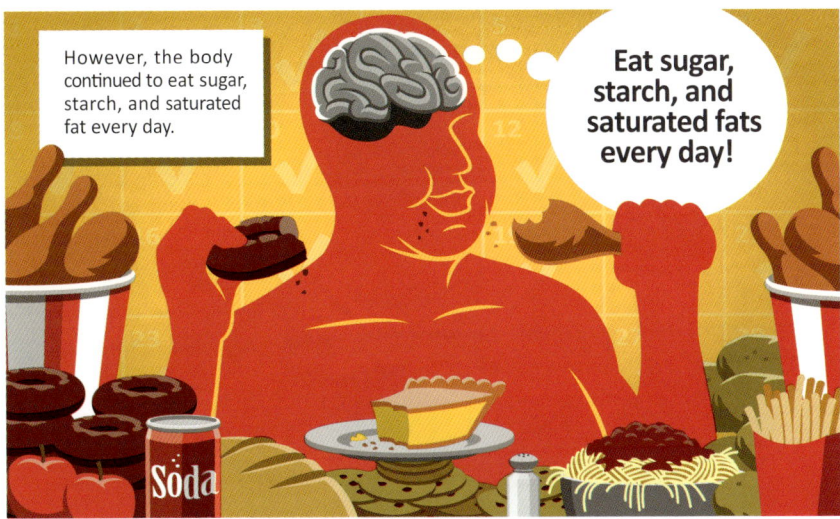

However, the body continued to eat sugar, starch, and saturated fat every day.

Eat sugar, starch, and saturated fats every day!

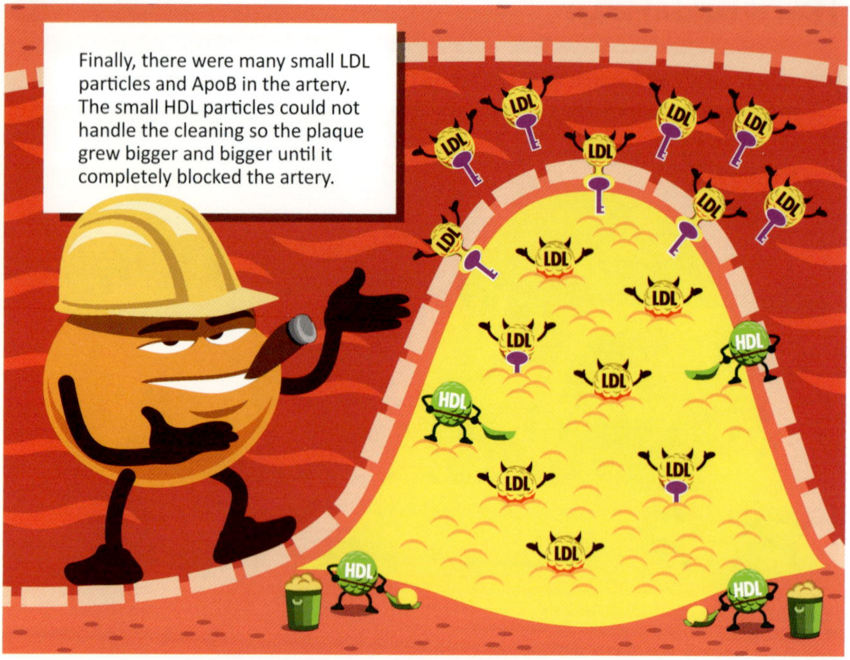

Finally, there were many small LDL particles and ApoB in the artery. The small HDL particles could not handle the cleaning so the plaque grew bigger and bigger until it completely blocked the artery.

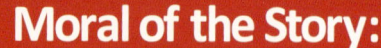

Moral of the Story:

If you don't want to increase LDL cholesterol, do not eat saturated fat.

If you don't want to increase ApoB, do not eat sugar and starch.

If you don't want to make LDL particles small in size, do not eat sugar and starch.

If you don't want to decrease ApoA-1 and HDL size, do not eat sugar and starch.

If you don't want to build plaque in your artery...

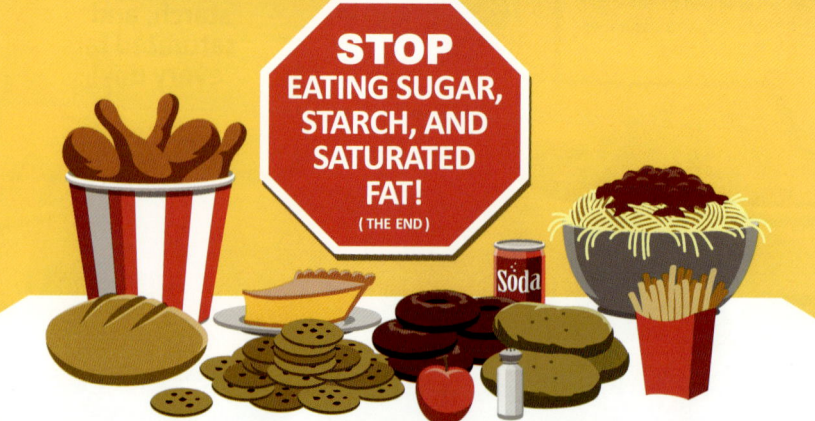

STOP
EATING SUGAR, STARCH, AND SATURATED FAT!
(THE END)

3

ratios

Ratios are comparisons of two numbers.

Several studies are now looking at ratios of different tests that have been proven to be valuable in assessing your heart disease risk.

These are not shown in your Health Diagnostic Laboratory, Inc. report. You have to make simple computations to find these out. We get the ratio by dividing the two test results being compared. Let's try it!

Total Cholesterol/HDL-C

The total cholesterol to HDL cholesterol ratio is a number that is helpful in predicting an individual's risk of developing atherosclerosis.

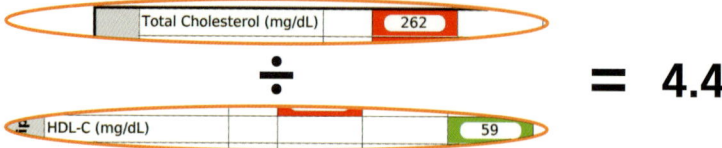

The number is obtained by dividing the total cholesterol value by the value of the HDL cholesterol. (High ratios indicate higher risk of a heart attack; low ratios indicate lower risk.)

High total cholesterol and low HDL cholesterol increases the ratio, and is undesirable. Conversely, high HDL cholesterol and low total cholesterol lowers the ratio and is desirable.

An average ratio would be about 4.5. Ideally you want to be better than average to prevent and reverse heart disease.

Your goal should be LESS THAN 2.5.

How can you decrease the Total Cholesterol/HDL-C ratio?

You can decrease this ratio by lowering your total cholesterol and increasing your HDL cholesterol, which you can achieve by eliminating sugar, starch, and saturated fat from your diet.

Triglycerides/HDL-C

HDL cholesterol is closely related to triglycerides. Researchers have found that it is common for people with high triglycerides to have low HDL cholesterol, which puts them at high risk for heart disease. The triglycerides/HDL-C ratio is one of the most potent predictors of heart disease.

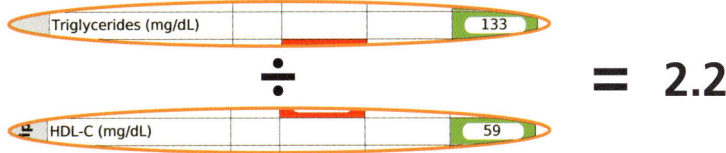

Triglycerides (mg/dL)   133

$\div$ $= 2.2$

HDL-C (mg/dL)   59

The number is obtained by dividing the triglyceride value by the value of the HDL cholesterol. The higher your triglycerides/HDL-C ratio, the more likely you will be to have a heart attack. In one study, those with the highest ratio were 16 times more at risk than those with the lowest ratio.

Your goal should be LESS THAN 2.

How can you improve your Triglycerides/HDL-C ratio?

You can improve your triglycerides/HDL-C ratio by eliminating sugar and starch from your diet. The speed at which simple changes in the diet can improve your triglycerides/HDL-C ratio was demonstrated in a study conducted by Gerald Reaven at Stanford, in which patients were put on diets consisting of the same number of calories but different protein-to-carbohydrate ratios. When these patients consumed a high-carbohydrate diet, they had a much higher triglycerides/HDL-C ratio than when they switched to a lower-carbohydrate diet. These changes occurred within four weeks of each dietary change.

ApoB/ApoA-1

The apoB/apoA-1 ratio has been shown to be the strongest single lipoprotein-related predictor of heart disease. While apoB plays a significant role in delivering cholesterol to tissue cells to form plaque, apoA-1 plays a major role in removing this cholesterol from plaque and disposing it to the liver. The apoB/apoA-1 ratio, therefore, represents a net balance between plaque-forming and plaque-cleaning lipoprotein particles.

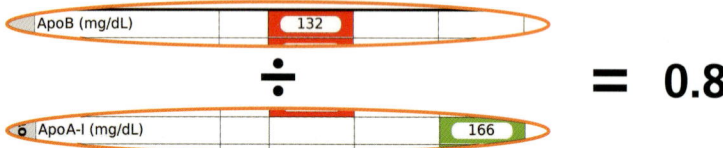

The number is obtained by dividing the apoB value by the value of the apoA-1. The higher your apoB/apoA-1 ratio, the more at risk you are of developing heart disease.

Your goal should be LESS THAN 0.5.

How can you decrease the apoB/apoA-1 ratio?

You can decrease this ratio by lowering your apoB and increasing your apoA-1, which you can achieve by eliminating sugar and starch from your diet.

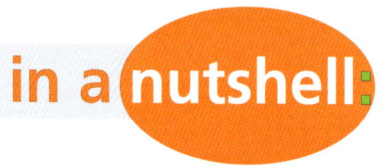

Low Ratio = Low Risk

Ratio	How to Lower
Total Cholesterol/HDL-C	Avoid sugar, starch, and saturated fat
Triglycerides/HDL-C	Avoid sugar and starch
ApoB/ApoA-1	Avoid sugar and starch

RECOMMENDATION: Learn more about sugar, starch, and saturated fat and how to avoid them by reading the book *Eat This, Lose That* by Kota J. Reddy, M.D. (available at www.reddybread.com).

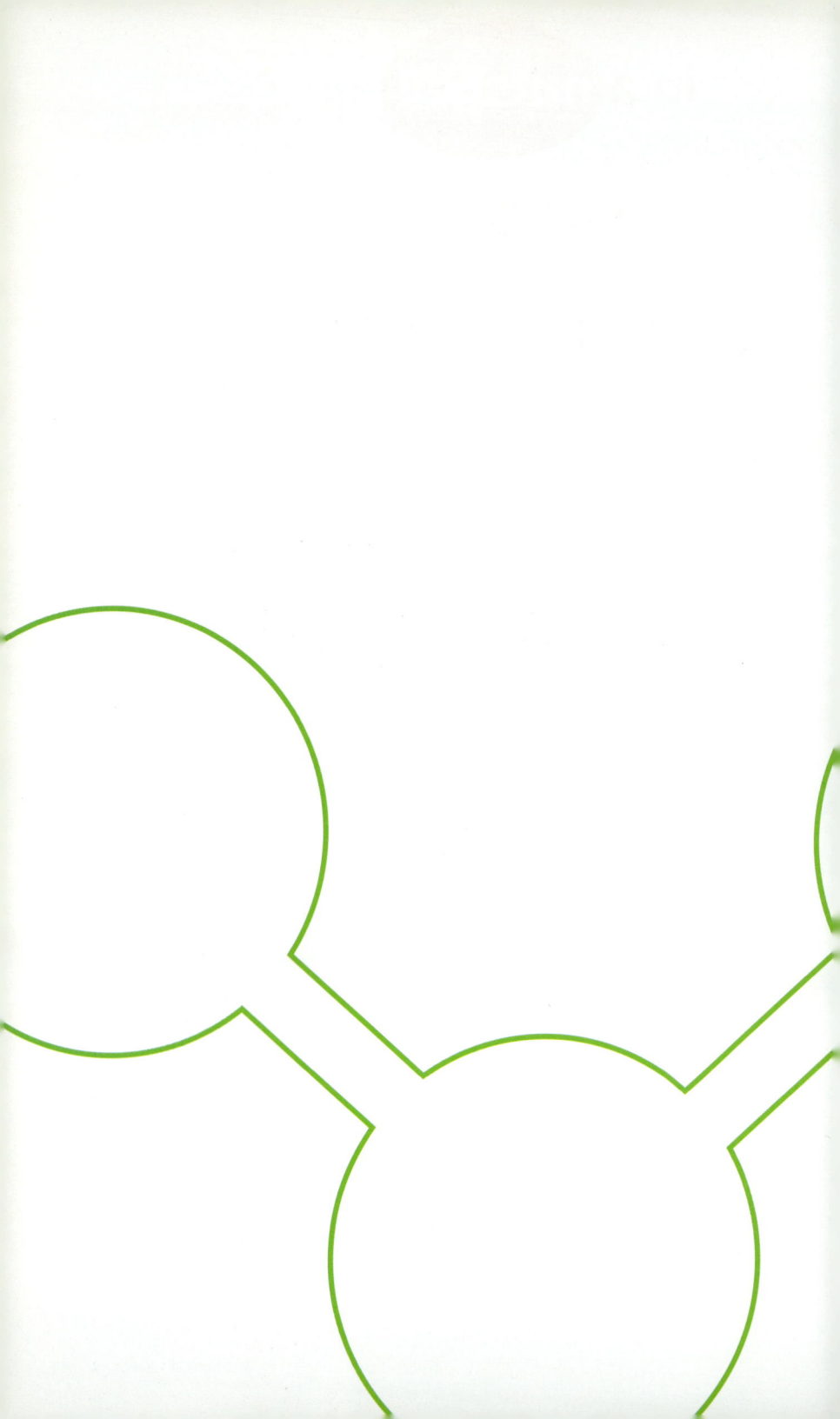

4

lipoprotein genetics

Everyone inherits many characteristics from their mother and father.

Some characteristics are beneficial, but others can be harmful. In the case of coronary heart disease, specific traits have been identified that can increase the risk of developing heart disease.

The most common gene affecting cholesterol levels is apolipoprotein E, or apoE. This is the trait that determines how your body processes cholesterol and how it responds to dietary fat, alcohol, exercise, and medications. It has three major variations: E2, E3, and E4. Individuals inherit one of these forms from each of their parents and thus have two copies. For example, if you inherit E3 from both parents, you have a combination called E3/E3. If you inherit an E2 from one parent and an E3 from the other parent, your combination is E2/E3. Other possible combinations are E2/2, E2/4, E3/4, and E4/4.

Laboratory Test	Notes	High Risk	Intermediate Risk	Optimal	High Risk Range	Intermediate Risk Range	Optimal Range	Previous Results
Lipoprotein Genetics Apolipoprotein E Genotype*				3/3	Estimated Genotype Frequency: 2/2 (~1-2%), 2/3 (~15%), 2/4 (~1-2%), 3/3 (~55%), 3/4 (~25%), 4/4 (~1-2%)			

E3 is the most common (60% of the population) and considered the normal type. E2 and E4 are results of genetic mutation, a permanent change from the normal state of the gene. Simply put, if you have any one of these mutations, you inherited an abnormal gene.

It is valuable to know which apoE genotype you have because if your genes are any combination of E4, you are at significantly higher risk of having heart disease. Around 20% of the population has this type of apoE. Several studies have shown that E4s are associated with higher levels of LDL cholesterol and apoB, which are strong risk factors for heart disease. However, these studies also tell us that among this E4 group, a low-fat diet, avoidance of alcohol, and cholesterol-lowering medication (when needed) can effectively lower cholesterol levels and decrease the risk of heart disease. If you test as E4, it is important that you stick to a low-fat diet and avoid alcohol as much as possible to lessen your risk of heart disease.

Testing for apoE genotype was used primarily to guide physicians in creating diet and therapeutic programs for patients with certain genotypes that put them at higher risk for heart disease. However, as research on apoE developed further, it was found that the apoE test can also detect the risk of Alzheimer's disease, particularly the late-onset type that occurs sometime after the age of 60. This is true especially if you have the E4 genotype and have a family history of the disease. With only one E4, the risk is as high as 49%. With two E4s, the risk goes up to 90%.

Unfortunately, this information can cause a dilemma for a person. Just imagine what your reaction would be if you found out that you have at least a 50% chance of developing Alzheimer's disease anytime after your 60th birthday. Genetic testing must always involve thorough consideration and careful weighing of the possible benefits and risks or harmful consequences that might result from the test findings.

Testing for apoE genotype can help guide your physician in creating a treatment plan for you. However, it will also give you information about your risk for Alzheimer's disease. While this is true, you must understand that it is not a marker of the disease, since there is no disease yet. It is only a predisposition, a chance, and not a certainty. Although one third of all people with Alzheimer's disease have the E4 genotype, not all E4s will develop the disease. Some individuals with the E4 genotype will never develop Alzheimer's disease, while others with no E4 may develop the disease.

The same situation is true with smoking and lung cancer. Smoking increases a person's risk of developing lung cancer, yet some heavy smokers never get cancer, while some nonsmokers do.

E2, on the other hand, is quite rare. It occurs in less than 10% of the population. Among them, only a few develop abnormal levels of cholesterol. Like E4s, these people may benefit from a low-fat, low-sugar diet and cholesterol medication.

Since apoE genotype is a fixed characteristic, it need only be tested once on an individual. This information guides your doctor on how to approach your treatment if you have abnormal cholesterol levels. The different apoE genotypes determine the success of diet and drug therapy.

ApoE Genotypes

	E2	E3	E4
Heart Disease Risk	Moderate Risk	Low Risk	High Risk
Low-Fat Diet	Decreases LDL-C (1x)	Decreases LDL-C (2x)	Decreases LDL-C (3x)
Moderate Alcohol	Decreases LDL-C Increases HDL-C	Increases HDL-C	Increases LDL-C Slightly Increases HDL-C (less so than E2 or E3)
Medications (Statins)	May Benefit	May Benefit	May Benefit
Alzheimer's Risk	Low Risk	Low Risk	High Risk

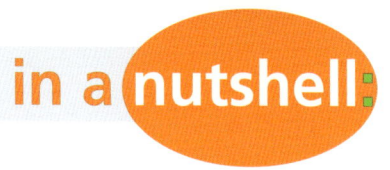

Summary of Key Lipoprotein Risk Markers

There are three important lipoprotein biomarkers you need to look at in your Health Diagnostic Laboratory, Inc. report:

1. LDL Particle Size

People with a lot of small LDL particles have a threefold risk of developing heart disease. Remember, diet high in sugar and starch make the bad cholesterol particles smaller in size.

2. Lp(a)

Lp(a) is also an inherited factor that increases risk of heart attack by as much as 70%. It is not affected by diet and exercise. Only niacin is proven to lower its concentration.

3. ApoE

If you have the 4/4 or 3/4 genotype, you are certainly at high risk for developing heart disease and possibly Alzheimer's disease. Avoiding sugar, starch, and saturated fat in the diet, abstinence from alcohol, and taking cholesterol-lowering medication (when needed) can decrease your risk.

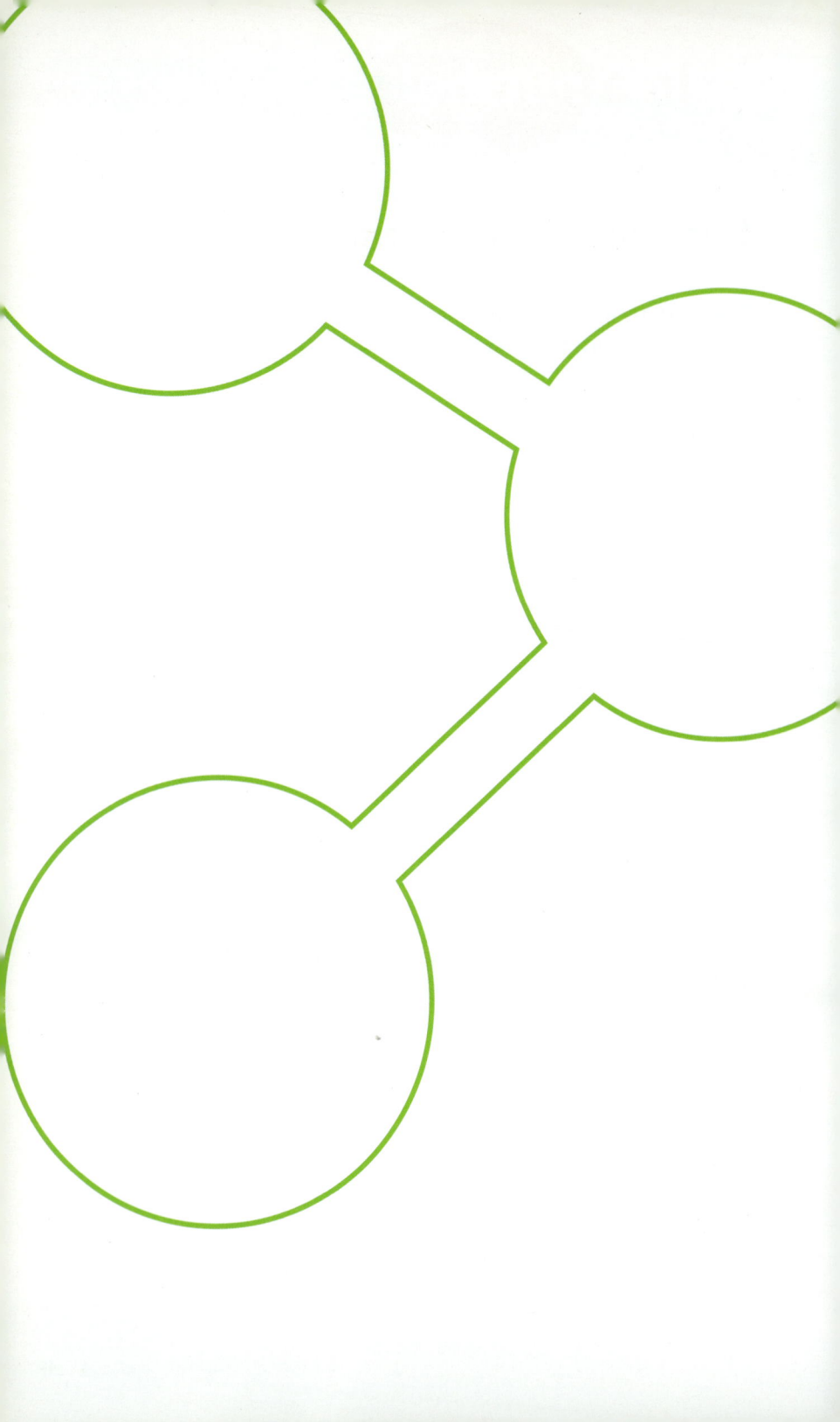

inflammatory markers

When tested as part of an advanced cholesterol profile, CRP (C-reactive protein) and fibrinogen are used mainly as markers of inflammation.

	Laboratory Test	Notes	High Risk	Intermediate Risk	Optimal	High Risk Range	Intermediate Risk Range	Optimal Range	Previous Results
Inflammation/ Oxidation	Myeloperoxidase (pmol/L)		718			≥ 550	400 - 549	< 400	
	Lp-PLA$_2$ (ng/mL)				193	≥ 235	200 - 234	< 200	
	hs-CRP (mg/L)		11.75			≥ 3.0	1.0 - 2.9	< 1.0	
	Fibrinogen (mg/dL)		550			≥ 465	301 - 464	< 300	

Inflammation is the body's natural reaction to infections, irritations, and other types of injury. Medical studies show that testing for these levels in the blood provides new ways to assess risk for heart disease.

CRP is a substance produced by the liver and fat cells. Its level dramatically rises when there is inflammation occurring in the body, including inflammation within the coronary arteries. In atherosclerosis, the higher the CRP, the greater the chance of a plaque rupturing and causing a heart attack. However, it is important to remember that CRP can also be high in other conditions such as infections, illnesses (like the "common cold" or flu), allergies, cancers, and arthritis. Therefore, if you have a high CRP level, other tests should be done to determine whether the inflammation is truly in the arteries of the heart. CRP only tells us that there is an inflammation in the body. It doesn't specifically point out where the inflammation is.

High CRP is Seen in Several Medical Conditions

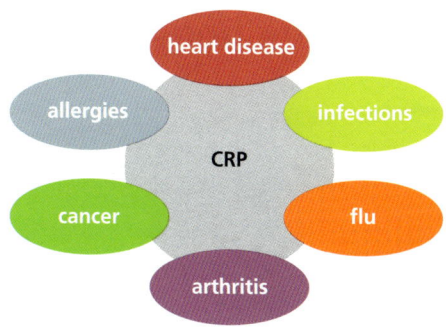

Fibrinogen is a sticky, fibrous protein substance that thickens the blood and promotes clotting that is part of the body's natural repair system. When there is tissue injury and inflammation in the arteries, the fibrinogen level rises as the body tries to repair the damage or stop a bleeding. However, the more fibrinogen there is, the thicker the blood, and the more the heart struggles to pump that thick blood to the whole body. There is also a greater chance of forming a clot that can obstruct an artery when the blood is too thick. Therefore, an increased level of fibrinogen puts a person at risk of developing heart disease and having a heart attack.

High levels of fibrinogen can also be caused by cigarette smoking, inactivity, aging, diabetes, and metabolic syndrome.

Your goal should be:

CRP	Less than 1.0
Fibrinogen	Less than 350

The lower the better!

Lipoprotein-associated phospholipase A2 or Lp-PLA$_2$ is another test that detects inflammation in the body.

Many years ago, atherosclerosis was thought to be caused mainly by an excessive deposit of cholesterol in the arteries. As a result, cholesterol became the focus of all heart disease prevention strategies. Now, it is becoming clearer that atherosclerosis is also an inflammatory disease and that inflammation plays a big role in its progression.

Whereas elevated CRP levels can indicate inflammation anywhere in the body, Lp-PLA$_2$ points specifically to inflammation of the coronary arteries; therefore, it is a predictor of heart attack and stroke.

	Laboratory Test	Notes	High Risk	Intermediate Risk	Optimal	High Risk Range	Intermediate Risk Range	Optimal Range	Previous Results
Inflammation/ Oxidation	Myeloperoxidase (pmol/L)		718			≥ 550	400 - 549	< 400	
	Lp-PLA$_2$ (ng/mL)				193	≥ 235	200 - 234	< 200	
	hs-CRP (mg/L)		11.75			≥ 3.0	1.0 - 2.9	< 1.0	
	Fibrinogen (mg/dL)		550			≥ 465	301 - 464	< 300	

Your goal should be LESS THAN 150.

Lp-PLA$_2$ is a substance that circulates in the bloodstream and likes to hang out with the bad cholesterol. Its presence in the plaque invites more LDL particles to come along and build up. It also triggers a process known as **oxidation**, which promotes inflammation within the artery. An elevated Lp-PLA$_2$ value indicates that the plaque is active.

To better understand this concept, let us draw an analogy to a volcano.

Dormant Volcano	Stable Plaque
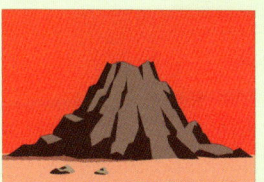	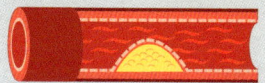

Dormant Volcano

Imagine a dormant volcano that has been sleeping for a long time.

Stable Plaque

Hard Plaque
- Large, blocks more than 50% of the artery
- Normal Lp-PLA₂ (no inflammation)
- Rarely ruptures
- Causes angina

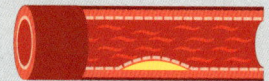

Soft Plaque
- Small, blocks less than 50% of the artery
- Normal Lp-PLA₂ (no inflammation)
- May not rupture (unless it becomes unstable with bad diet)

A stable plaque is like a dormant volcano sleeping. It may or may not give you symptoms, depending on the type of plaque, but it will not erupt at anytime.

Active Volcano

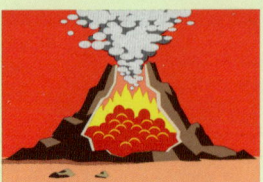

Suddenly, hot molten lava starts building up inside the volcano. The once silent and sleeping mountain now awakens and starts showing smoke, signifying it is active.

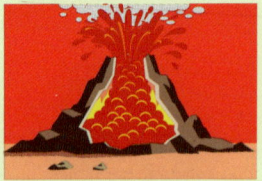

As the pressure inside increases further, the inevitable happens: The volcano erupts and brings about destruction.

Unstable Plaque

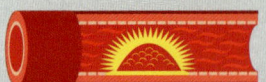

Unstable Plaque

A diet high in sugar, starch, and saturated fat increases Lp-PLA₂ within the plaque and awakens it. Inflammation sets in.

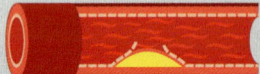

As the inflammation increases, the cap covering the plaque starts to thin out, making it prone to breaking, until finally the plaque ruptures and causes a potentially fatal heart attack.

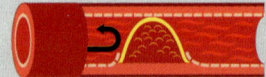

High Lp-PLA$_2$ is a sign that there is a plaque somewhere in the arteries that is ready to crack and cause a heart attack or stroke.

Unfortunately, there is no way of detecting if a plaque is ready to rupture. No imaging test can show this, and you will not even have any symptoms. That is why it is important to know your level of Lp-PLA$_2$, so you can do something if it is high. High Lp-PLA$_2$ is a sign that there is a plaque somewhere in the arteries that is ready to crack and cause a heart attack or stroke. Controlling your blood pressure, proper diet (eliminate sugars, starches, saturated fats in your diet), exercise, reducing stress, and taking fish oils have been shown to lower Lp-PLA$_2$ levels.

Your goal should be
LESS THAN 150ng/ml.
(preferably <100ng/ml)

What increases your Lp-PLA$_2$?

A diet rich in sugar, starch, and saturated fat will increase Lp-PLA$_2$ level. A sudden increase in your Lp-PLA$_2$ tells you that your diet for the past six months has been high in sugar, starch, and saturated fat. Now, you have an increased inflammation in your arterial wall. It signifies that somewhere there is a plaque ready to rupture and cause a heart attack or stroke.

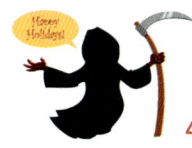

40% increase in heart attacks!

JAN	FEB	MAR	APR	MAY	JUN	JUL	AUG	SEP	OCT	NOV	D	Dec. 16 thru Jan. 15

————————— 60% —————————   ——— holiday season ———

If you want to decrease Lp-PLA$_2$ and your risk for heart attack and stroke, avoid foods with a combination of either sugar and saturated fat or starch and saturated fat.

This could be one of the reasons why there has been a 40% increase in heart attacks happening in the last two weeks of December and first two weeks of January. The relative change in diet starting in Halloween, followed by Thanksgiving, Christmas, and New Year's could explain the elevations in inflammatory markers. During these holidays, foods high in sugar and starch, such as cookies, chocolates, ice cream, and other desserts, are readily available.

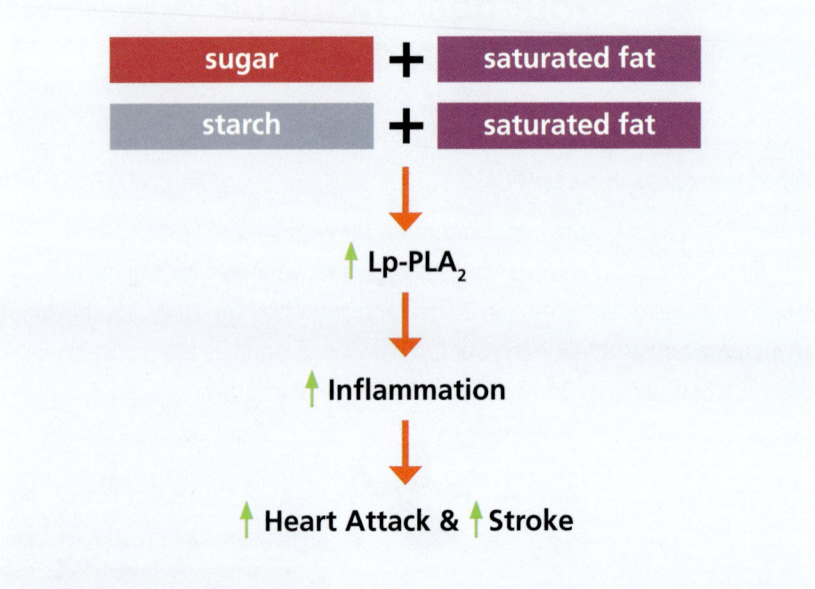

Myeloperoxidase, or MPO, is an enzyme made by white blood cells (WBCs), the body's defenses during times of injury and infection.

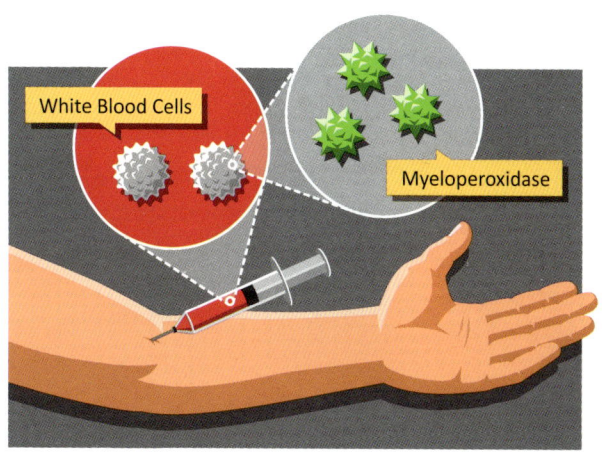

MPO is part of WBCs' artillery. It produces oxidants and free radicals to ward off infections and mobilize cells to repair damaged tissues.

Laboratory Test	Notes	High Risk	Intermediate Risk	Optimal	High Risk Range	Intermediate Risk Range	Optimal Range	Previous Results
Myeloperoxidase (pmol/L)		718			≥ 550	400 - 549	< 400	
Lp-PLA₂ (ng/mL)				193	≥ 235	200 - 234	< 200	
hs-CRP (mg/L)		11.75			≥ 3.0	1.0 - 2.9	< 1.0	
Fibrinogen (mg/dL)		550			≥ 465	201 - 464	< 200	

Unfortunately, these substances can also damage the endothelium (inner lining of blood vessels). MPO consumes **nitric oxide,** the substance that maintains the health of endothelial cells. Low levels of nitric oxide cause dysfunction of the endothelial lining, which is the starting point of heart disease and other metabolic diseases (like diabetes). Furthermore, MPO oxidizes LDLs (the bad cholesterol carriers), which makes them a greater risk factor. Endothelial dysfunction plus cholesterol gone bad is the perfect formula to promote plaque formation and heart disease.

MPO is linked to inflammation and heart disease. A high level of the enzyme predicts an early risk of a heart attack. Although MPO is not a routine test, it must be part of a complete workup for a patient who is at risk of a heart attack, especially when inflammatory markers are high, such as Lp-PLA$_2$.

What can increase your MPO level?

A diet high in sugar, starch, and saturated fat can increase your MPO level, thus increasing your risk for inflammation and heart attack. Studies have also shown that foods high in fructose and smoking can increase this inflammatory marker.

Your goal should be LESS THAN 400.

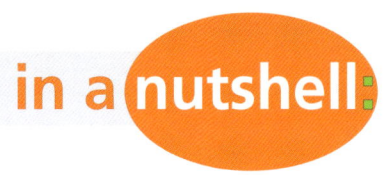

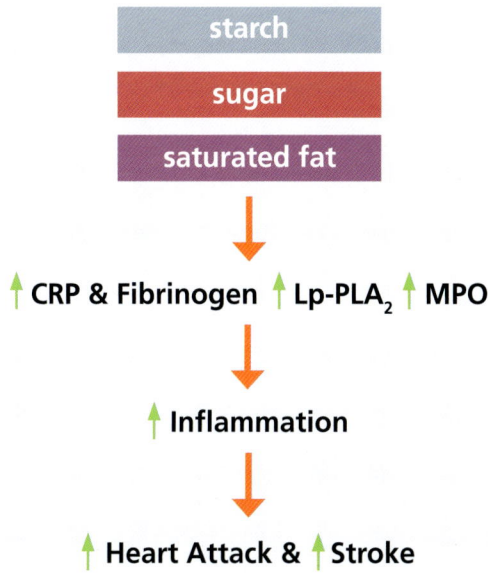

If you want to decrease the inflammation in your arteries and your risk for heart attack and stroke, avoid foods with sugar, starch, and saturated fat.

RECOMMENDATION: Learn more about sugar, starch, and saturated fat and how to avoid them by reading the book *Eat This, Lose That* by Kota J. Reddy, M.D. (available at www.reddybread.com).

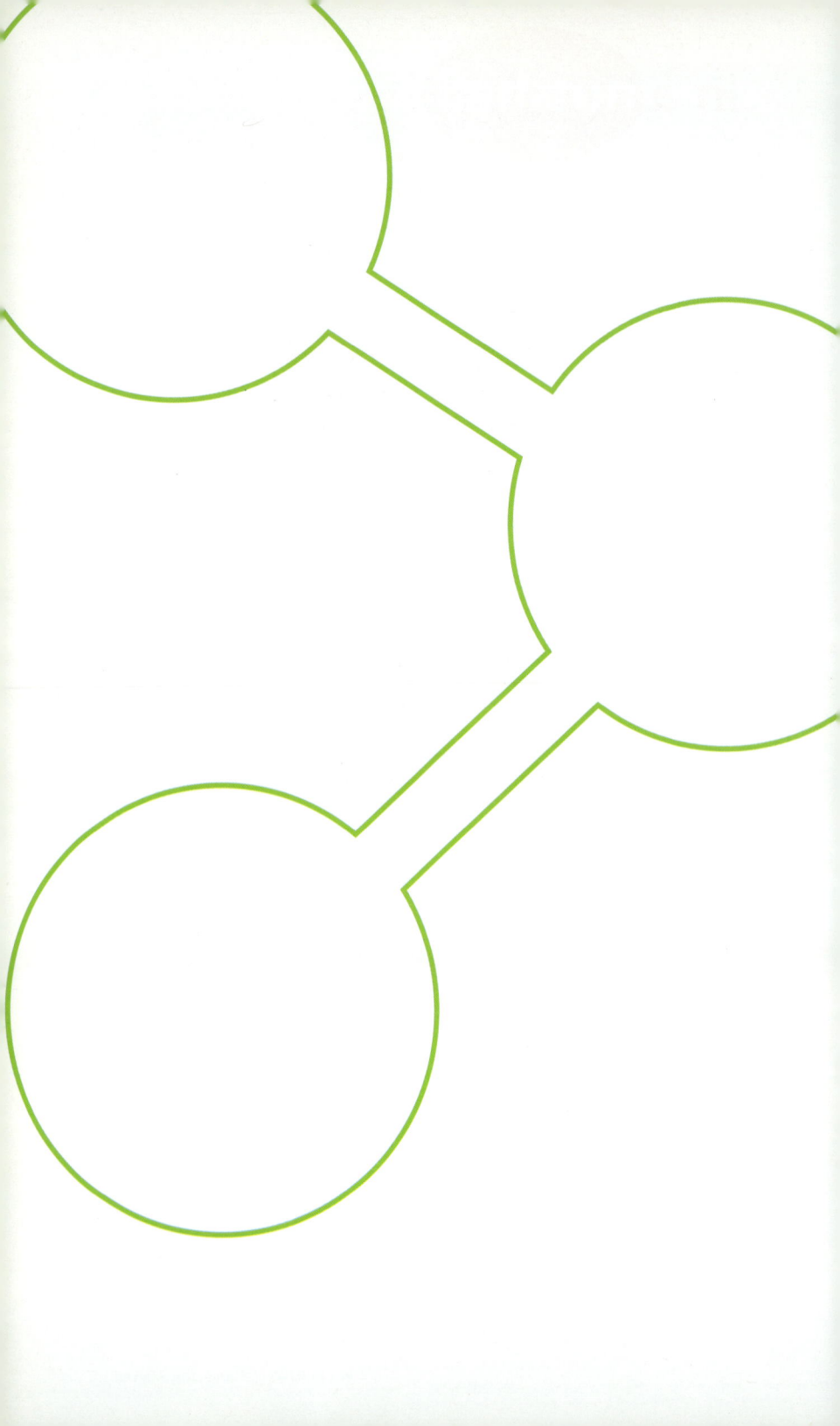

6

myocardial stress

Other causes of heart failure are as follows:

Condition	Reason
Heart valve disease	May result from diseases, infections (endocarditis) or a defect at birth. Blood may leak back through a defective valve causing the heart to work harder to keep the blood moving. Workload increases, which results in heart failure.
Anemia (low hemoglobin)	When there are low red blood cells (RBCs) to carry oxygen, the heart works double time to send these limited cells to the body.
Cardiomyopathy (heart muscle disease)	Any damage to the heart muscles (whether due to drugs, alcohol abuse, or viral infections) can lead to heart failure. Also seen in patients with AICD and/or pacemaker.
Diabetes	It increases the risk for CAD and hypertension.
Thyroid disease (both hypo- and hyperthyroidism)	Hypo: weakens the heart. Hyper: makes the heart work at a faster rate.
Too much salt intake	Salt causes water retention; therefore, it increases blood pressure and workload of the heart.
Cancer treatment (radiation or chemo)	It is toxic to the heart.
Alcohol abuse	It leads to cardiomyopathy.
Pulmonary Hypertension	Increases stress on the heart.
Renal Failure	Increases stress on the heart.
Atrial Fibrillation	If uncorrected may lead to heart failure. Patients with atrial fibrillation were found to have high NT-proBNP level.
Sleep apnea	It causes right-sided heart failure.

Bear in mind that some of these conditions can be present without your awareness. Having more than one of these factors dramatically increases your risk. Anything that causes heart failure can increase your NT-proBNP; therefore, it is also important to include a NT-proBNP test in your heart disease prevention plan because it can detect conditions, of which you may not even be aware, that could be damaging your heart.

Note on Sleep Apnea:

Sleep apnea is a sleep disorder wherein your breathing stops or gets very shallow and your lungs are not getting enough air or oxygen. This can happen repeatedly during the entire duration of sleep, sometimes hundreds of times during the night and often lasting from 30 seconds to more than a minute.

There are two types of sleep apnea: **obstructive apnea** and **central apnea.** The obstructive type is the most common. It results in numerous interruptions to breathing caused by a blockage in the airway or windpipe. It may be blocked by the tongue, tonsils, or uvula (the little piece of flesh that hangs down in the back of the throat) as they collapse backward during sleep when throat muscles become relaxed. It may also be blocked by a large amount of fatty tissue in the throat especially in people who are overweight or obese.

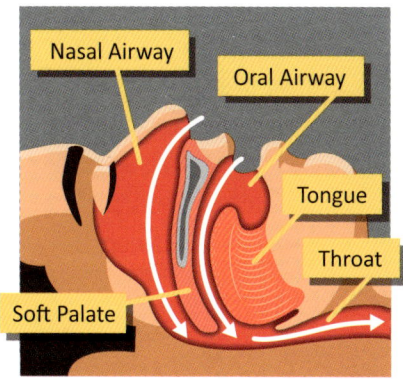
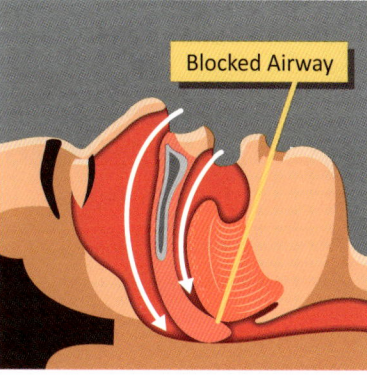

When you try to breathe through a narrowed airway, you will produce loud snoring caused by the vibration of the relaxed throat. This could be annoying especially if you share your bed with someone. Snoring is an indication that you could be having obstructive sleep apnea (OSA). It is associated with frequent wake-ups from sleep. Most of the time you won't even remember waking up, but it disturbs your sleep and results in a poor quality of rest. That is why people with OSA experience excessive tiredness and sleepiness during the day.

Central sleep apnea (CSA), on the other hand, is rare. With this type of sleep apnea, the problem lies in the "drive" to breathe. There is usually insufficient drive to breathe when the breathing center of the brain is damaged due to either stroke or trauma. When this happens, the brain fails to transmit signals to the respiratory muscles (muscles for breathing), so breathing is halted. A direct damage to the respiratory muscles by conditions such as multiple sclerosis can also cause this breathing problem. People with CSA will periodically stop breathing as they lose their drive to breathe.

If sleep apnea is left untreated, it could lead to a lot of serious health problems. Of more concern is its effect on cardiovascular health. We are now finding out that many deaths among people in their 40s and over, which are attributed to heart disease, may actually be related to sleep apnea.

When you stop breathing during sleep, your oxygen level drops. The brain senses this as a danger because it cannot survive without oxygen. It thinks that there is not enough blood flowing to its territory to supply the needed oxygen, so it tells the body to release an adrenaline-like substance into the bloodstream that will increase the blood pressure to compensate and return the normal blood flow to the brain. If sleep apnea becomes persistent, the high blood pressure becomes sustained and may not return to a normal level. This is when it all goes downhill for your heart.

The changes in blood pressure may increase the risk for heart failure. When blood pressure is high, the heart has to work harder and this causes damage to its muscles. Heartbeats may also become uncoordinated, which causes arrhythmias or rhythm problems. The most common is atrial fibrillation. This occurs when the two upper chambers of the heart (atria) beat irregularly and out of synchronicity with the two lower chambers (ventricles). Finally, high blood pressure can directly damage the lining of the arteries (endothelium) through shear stress. As a result, the artery becomes prone to fatty buildup and develops coronary artery disease.

Sleep apnea may be linked to several other conditions such as impotence, obesity, drowsiness, fatigue, diabetes, headache, stroke, lung hypertension, and dementia or memory loss. Untreated sleep apnea may also be responsible for job impairment and motor vehicular accidents.

Problems Linked to Sleep Apnea

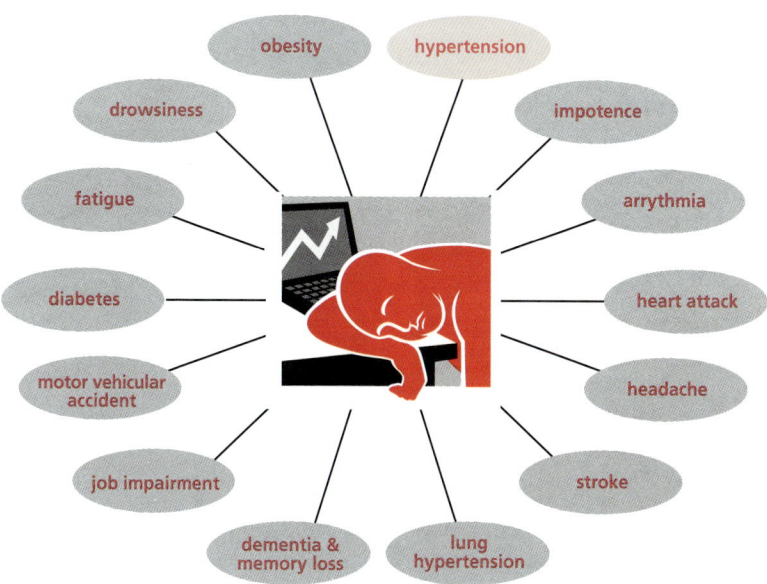

Sleep apnea is more common than we previously thought. According to the National Institutes of Health, it affects more than 12 million Americans. The most common risk factors for sleep apnea include male gender and being overweight. Although it is common among people over the age of 40, sleep apnea can strike anyone at any age, even children. Unfortunately, the general public still lacks awareness and health care professionals have not adopted a routine medical practice to recognize sleep apnea in patients who are at risk. The vast majority remain undiagnosed, and therefore untreated, despite the fact that this serious disorder has dangerous consequences.

A NT-proBNP level greater than 125 but less than 450 could be seen in obstructive sleep apnea and pulmonary hypertension. If the heart function is normal and the NT-proBNP level is on the high side, always check for sleep apnea.

The approved treatment for sleep apnea is called **Continuous Positive Airway Pressure** or CPAP. It is a specialized mask that you wear while you sleep. It is connected to a small machine that delivers additional pressure to the air you breathe. By doing so, it helps keep the airway open at all times.

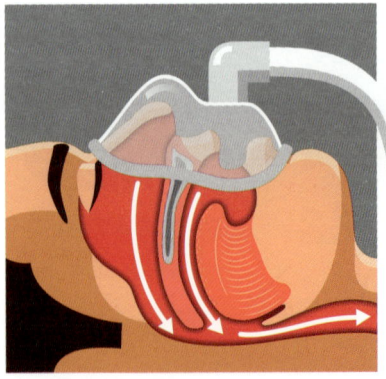
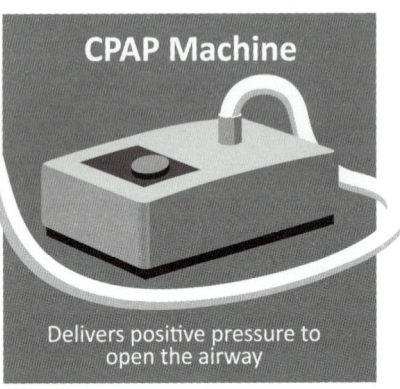

CPAP Machine

Delivers positive pressure to open the airway

Rarely, surgery would be necessary to correct obstructive sleep apnea. Common procedures include removing the tonsils and extra tissues from the throat to relieve the obstruction.

Lifestyle modifications such as avoiding sleep medications and alcohol before bedtime can also help reduce the occurrence of sleep apnea. Alcohol and sleep medications relax and make the muscles of your throat collapse backward when you lie down, thereby obstructing your airway. Quitting smoking, losing weight, and sleeping on your side are other lifestyle modifications you can try to prevent sleep apnea.

Sleep apnea can be treated. The key is to recognize its presence early by identifying warning signs and symptoms as they appear. Ask your physician today if you are at risk and find out if you need to have a sleep study to check if you have sleep apnea.

If you (or someone you know) have one or more of the following symptoms, you probably have sleep apnea and need a sleep study.

- Snoring
- Problem sleeping (insomnia) or restless sleep
- Gasping for breath or choking, after a pause in breathing
- Daytime sleepiness
- Morning headaches
- Fatigue, loss of energy
- Sexual dysfunction (e.g., impotence, lack of desire)
- Forgetfulness or trouble concentrating
- Irritability or mood changes
- Anxiety or depression
- Overweight
- Large neck size
- High blood pressure
- Drowsy while driving
- Waking up with a dry mouth
- Frequent leg jerks/movements or restless legs
- Heartburn
- Frequent trips to the bathroom at night
- Excessive night sweating

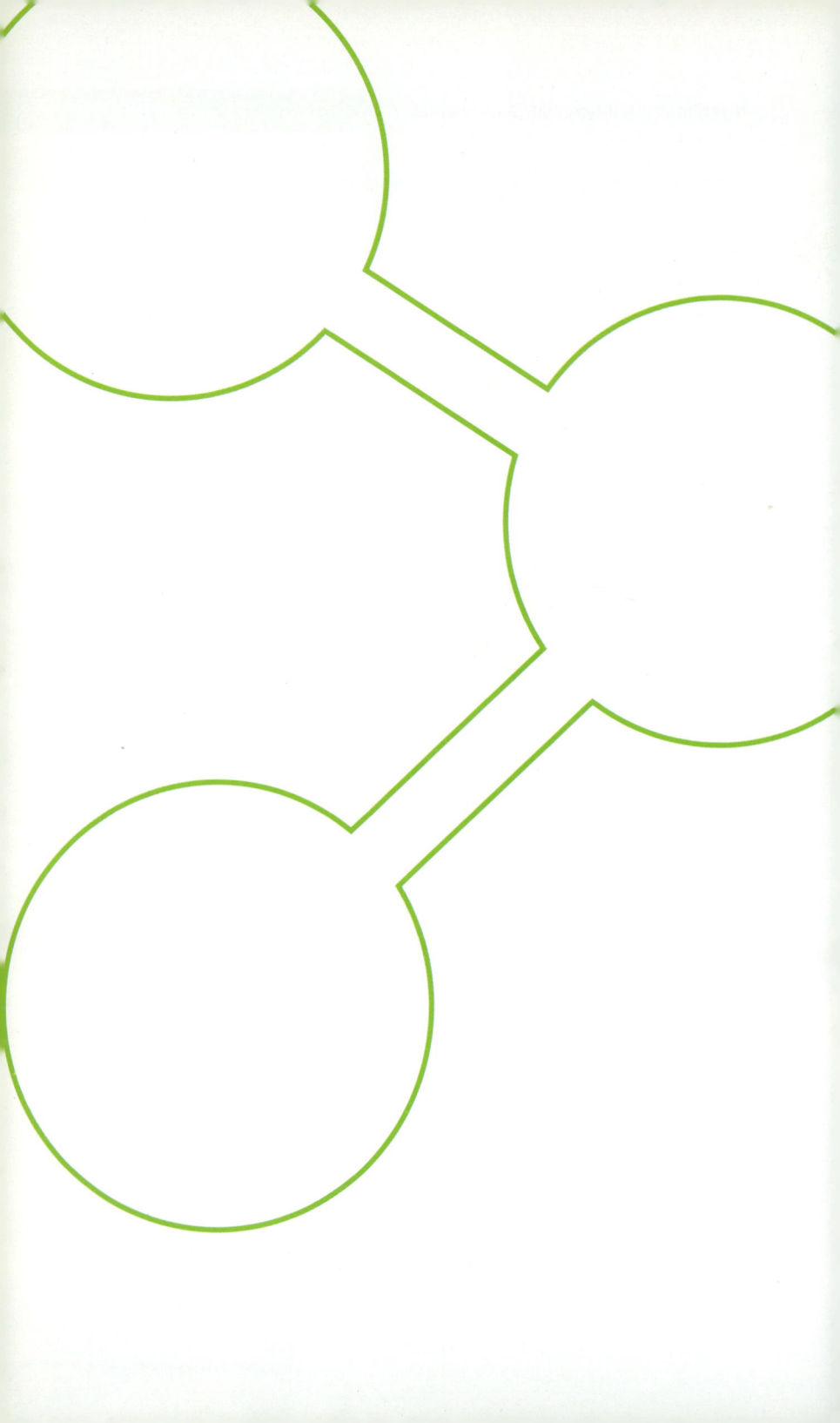

7

other metabolic tests

Laboratory Test	Notes	High Risk	Intermediate Risk	Optimal	High Risk Range	Intermediate Risk Range	Optimal Range	Previous Results
Insulin (µU/mL)				3	≥ 12	10 - 11	3 - 9	
Free Fatty Acid (mmol/L)		1.05			> 0.7	0.6 - 0.7	≤ 0.59	
Glucose (mg/dL)		286			≤ 55 or > 125	56-69 or 100-125	70 - 99	
HbA1c (%)				6.3	≥ 6.5	6.0 - 6.4	4.8 - 5.9	
25-hydroxy-Vitamin D (ng/mL)		12			≤ 14	15 - 29	30 - 100	
Uric Acid (mg/dL)				7.2	≥ 8	7.0 - 7.9	3.4 - 6.9	
TSH (µIU/mL)				0.79	< 0.27 or > 4.20		0.27 - 4.20	
Homocysteine (µmol/L)								

Our body's main source of energy is in the form of glucose or blood sugar.

We get most of it from digesting carbohydrates in our diet. Foods like rice, pasta, grains, potatoes, fruits, some vegetables, and processed sweets are broken down into glucose by our digestive system. It then gets absorbed through the small intestine and into the bloodstream.

In the blood, glucose is met by a hormone known as **insulin**—a hormone secreted by the pancreas to regulate blood glucose. Insulin stimulates all of the cells in your body, especially in your muscles and liver, to open up, take in glucose, and use it as energy for their daily functions. This is the body's way of burning calories.

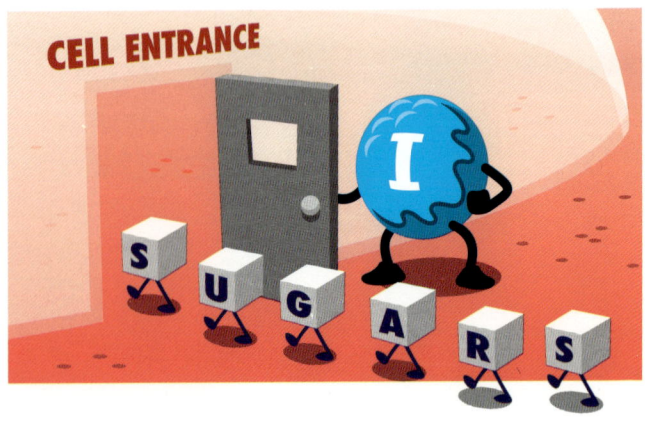

The pancreas is stimulated to produce and secrete insulin, depending on the level of blood glucose. When your glucose level is high, it could be a sign that you may have more sugar than you presently need. Your body is not burning the sugar, and therefore, it is accumulating in the blood. Your body senses this and releases more insulin to stimulate the liver and muscles to take in more glucose and store it for future use in chains called **glycogen.**

Conversely, if glucose is in short supply and food is unavailable, the pancreas stops secreting insulin and, instead, releases a different type of hormone called **glucagon.** This hormone makes the liver and muscles break down glycogen stores and releases glucose into the bloodstream to replenish glucose supply. The key is to maintain a normal blood glucose level. There is always a low level of insulin being secreted to maintain a constant glucose concentration in the blood.

When you eat a lot of sugars and starches, the so-called **high-glycemic carbohydrates,** you flood your blood with excess glucose. Your body reacts by releasing more insulin. If you can't burn all the sugar, it will be stored as glycogen. However, you can only store a small amount of glycogen at a time. Once your glycogen reserve is full, the leftover sugar gets stored as fat. This is what creates belly fat. Too much belly fat increases your risk for inflammation and heart attack.

Your goal should be:

Glucose	80 to 90mg/dL (before meals)
Insulin	3 to 11 µU/ml

Having high insulin all the time is also bad. It is toxic to the body and causes several problems, including hypertension. Insulin makes you retain sodium and water, which makes your blood pressure high and increases your risk for heart failure. People with high insulin are also likely to have high levels of homocysteine, a substance that can increase your risk of heart disease and strokes. More importantly, when our cells are constantly exposed to high levels of insulin, they develop resistance to it. Cells are thought to become insulin resistant because they are trying to protect themselves from the toxic effect of insulin.

As the body becomes immune to the effects of insulin, the blood sugar rises, and the pancreas compensates by releasing more insulin, thus increasing the resistance further. This becomes a vicious cycle, and the person develops **Insulin resistance syndrome**, also known as **Metabolic Syndrome** or **Syndrome X**. This syndrome includes a consistent high level of insulin, abdominal obesity (lots of belly fat), high blood pressure, and abnormalities in cholesterol (increased number of small LDLs, low amount of HDLs and high triglycerides), which promote plaque formation in the arteries. Insulin resistance increases your risk for several chronic diseases, such heart disease, obesity, diabetes, and cancers.

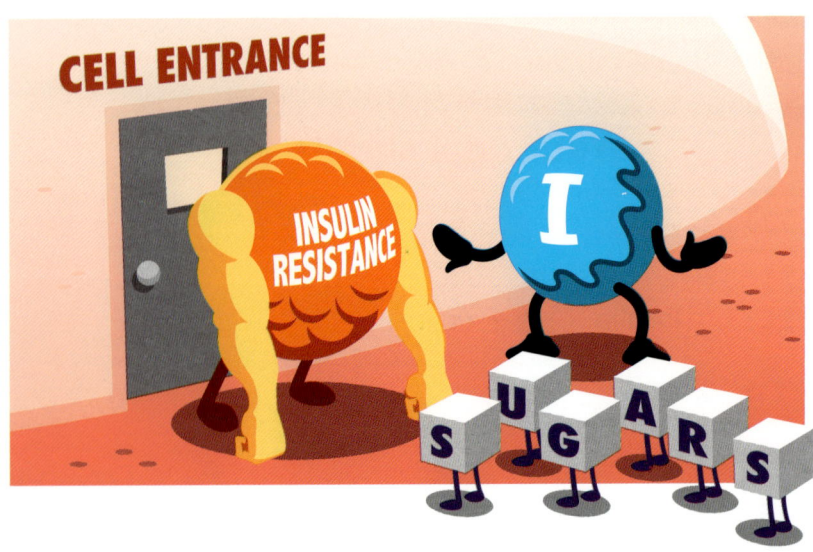

Excessive eating of sugar and starch is the primary culprit in the development of insulin resistance. Eliminating these in your diet is the best way to stop its progression. Interestingly, exercise has been found to help people with insulin resistance in controlling their sugar levels. Exercise is thought to stimulate cells to open up and let glucose in without the need for insulin. This explains why a person's blood sugar drops after exercising.

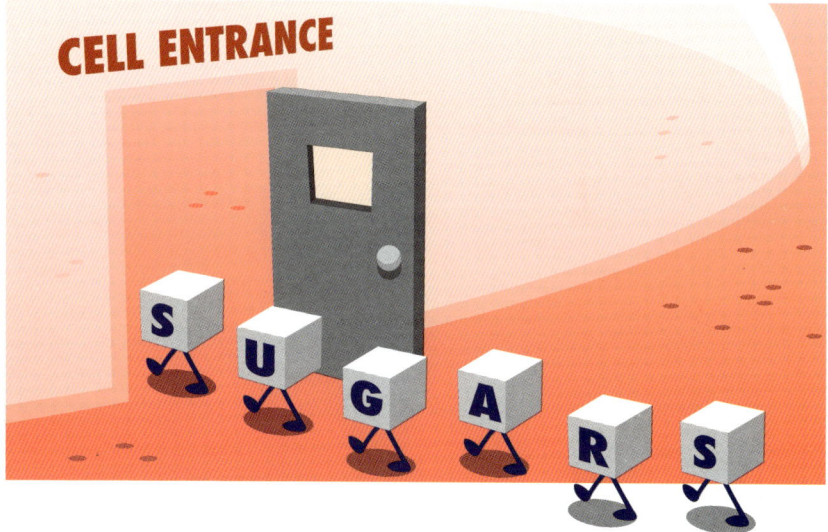

Exercise opens the doors of cells without the need for insulin.

Hemoglobin A1c (HbA1c) or **glycated hemoglobin** is a test that determines how much your blood glucose has been controlled for the last three to four months.

Laboratory Test	Notes	High Risk	Intermediate Risk	Optimal	High Risk Range	Intermediate Risk Range	Optimal Range	Previous Results
Insulin (µU/mL)				3	≥ 12	10 - 11	3 - 9	
Free Fatty Acid (mmol/L)		1.05			> 0.7	0.6 - 0.7	≤ 0.59	
Glucose (mg/dL)		286			≤ 55 or > 125	56-69 or 100-125	70 - 99	
HbA1c (%)			6.3		≥ 6.5	6.0 - 6.4	4.8 - 5.9	
25-hydroxy-Vitamin D (ng/mL)		12			≤ 14	15 - 29	30 - 100	
Uric Acid (mg/dL)			7.2		≥ 8	7.0 - 7.9	3.4 - 6.9	
TSH (µIU/mL)				0.79	< 0.27 or > 4.20		0.27 - 4.20	
Homocysteine (µmol/L)								

Your goal should be LESS THAN 5%.

This test is different from the regular blood glucose test or the finger stick measure of blood sugar that a person with diabetes does every day at home. Those tests only measure blood sugar at any given time. HbA1c gives a bigger picture. It summarizes your blood glucose level for the past three to four months. Think of it like a performance evaluation of your job. A single day's work doesn't give much for an assessment of your performance, does it? People with diabetes benefit from this test because it gives them an idea of how well their treatment is working.

Hemoglobin is a protein found inside the red blood cells (RBCs), and it carries oxygen to all other cells of the body. When you have too much sugar in your blood, the RBCs gobble it up, and it attaches to the hemoglobin inside. This process is called **glycation of hemoglobin.** The lifespan of a RBC is approximately 120 days. Glucose stays attached to hemoglobin for the entire life of the RBC, so if you test for HbA1c, it will reflect the glucose level over the past three to four months.

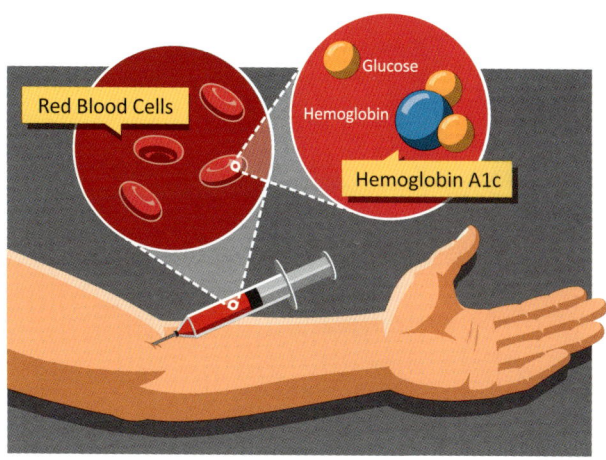

The normal range for HbA1c is between 4% and 6%. Higher values increase the risk of complications. Your goal should be less than 5%, which signifies a well-controlled sugar level.

There is a correlation between hemoglobin A1c levels and average blood sugar levels. The chart on the next page will be very helpful in illustrating this correlation. Use it to find your average blood glucose when you know your HbA1c. The chart is specially color-coded so you can easily interpret your level of health based on your HbA1c. If you check your glucose levels several times a day, you can also use this chart to predict your HbA1c for the next three to four months.

Keeping blood sugar at a normal range improves HbA1c. Studies have shown that for every 1% reduction in HbA1c, there is a 10% decrease in the risk of complications. If your HbA1c is 9.5% and you drop it to 7.5%, you reduce your risk by 20%, even if your HbA1c is still not within goal.

Hemoglobin A1C & Blood Sugar (glucose) Conversion Table

	EXCELLENT					GOOD				
HbA1c	4.0	4.1	4.2	4.3	4.4	4.5	4.6	4.7	4.8	4.9
Blood Sugar (MG/DL)	65	69	72	76	79	83	86	90	93	97

	SATISFACTORY					NEEDS IMPROVEMENT				
HbA1c	5.0	5.1	5.2	5.3	5.4	5.5	5.6	5.7	5.8	5.9
Blood Sugar (MG/DL)	101	104	108	111	115	118	122	126	129	133

	WARNING					DANGEROUS				
HbA1c	6.0	6.1	6.2	6.3	6.4	6.5	6.6	6.7	6.8	6.9
Blood Sugar (MG/DL)	136	140	143	147	151	154	158	161	165	168

	DANGEROUS									
HbA1c	7.0	7.1	7.2	7.3	7.4	7.5	7.6	7.7	7.8	7.9
Blood Sugar (MG/DL)	172	176	180	183	186	190	193	197	200	204

	VERY DANGEROUS									
HbA1c	8.0	8.1	8.2	8.3	8.4	8.5	8.6	8.7	8.8	8.9
Blood Sugar (MG/DL)	207	211	215	218	222	225	229	232	236	240

	DEADLY									
HbA1c	9.0	9.5	10.0	10.5	11.0	11.5	12.0	12.5	13.0	13.5
Blood Sugar (MG/DL)	243	261	279	297	314	332	350	368	386	403

Fatty acids are acids produced when fats are broken down. They are often used for energy by most types of cells in the body.

Fatty acids are usually bound or attached to other molecules. When they are not attached to other molecules, they are called "free" fatty acids.

Laboratory Test	Notes	High Risk	Intermediate Risk	Optimal	High Risk Range	Intermediate Risk Range	Optimal Range	Previous Results
Insulin (μU/mL)				3	≥ 12	10 - 11	3 - 9	
Free Fatty Acid (mmol/L)		1.05			> 0.7	0.6 - 0.7	≤ 0.59	
Glucose (mg/dL)		286			≤ 55 or > 125	56-69 or 100-125	70 - 99	
HbA1c (%)			6.3		≥ 6.5	6.0 - 6.4	4.8 - 5.9	
25-hydroxy-Vitamin D (ng/mL)		12			≤ 14	15 - 29	30 - 100	
Uric Acid (mg/dL)			7.2		≥ 8	7.0 - 7.9	3.4 - 6.9	
TSH (μIU/mL)				0.79	< 0.27 or > 4.20		0.27 - 4.20	
Homocysteine (μmol/L)								

This test is important because elevated free fatty acids are associated with metabolic syndrome. This syndrome includes a consistently high level of insulin, abdominal obesity (lots of belly fat), high blood pressure, and abnormalities in cholesterol (increased number of small LDLs, low amount of HDLs and high triglycerides), which promote plaque formation in the arteries.

People with metabolic syndrome are at risk for several chronic diseases, such as heart disease, obesity, diabetes, and cancers.

Metabolic Syndrome

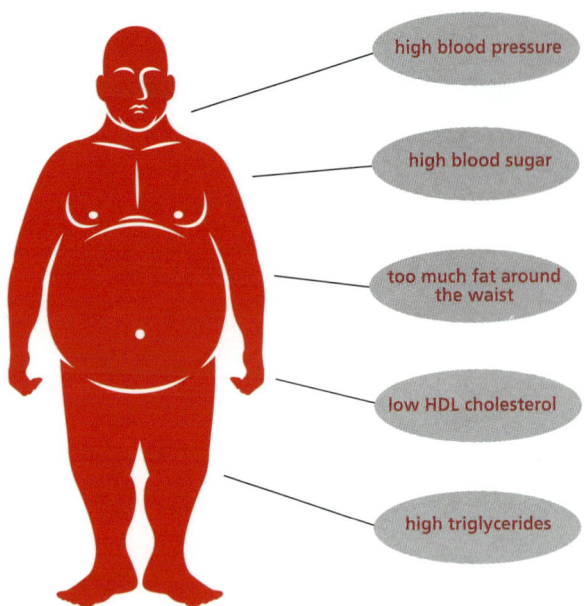

high blood pressure

high blood sugar

too much fat around the waist

low HDL cholesterol

high triglycerides

Elevated free fatty acid is a sign that you are at risk for developing adult-onset diabetes. Eliminating sugar, starch, and saturated fat in your diet along with increased exercise and weight loss can help lower free fatty acids.

Your goal should be LESS THAN 0.59.

Thyroid stimulating hormone (TSH) is the hormone released from the pituitary gland of the brain that stimulates the thyroid to release its hormones.

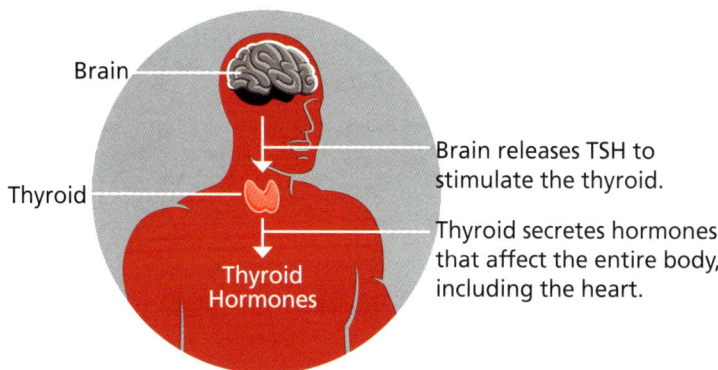

Brain

Thyroid

Thyroid Hormones

Brain releases TSH to stimulate the thyroid.

Thyroid secretes hormones that affect the entire body, including the heart.

Thyroid hormones control practically all of the body's functions. They at least have some effect on every organ in the body, including the heart. A blood test for TSH determines whether your thyroid is functioning properly.

Laboratory Test	Notes	High Risk	Intermediate Risk	Optimal	High Risk Range	Intermediate Risk Range	Optimal Range	Previous Results
Insulin (µU/mL)				3	≥ 12	10 - 11	3 - 9	
Free Fatty Acid (mmol/L)		1.05			> 0.7	0.6 - 0.7	≤ 0.59	
Glucose (mg/dL)		286			≤ 55 or > 125	56-69 or 100-125	70 - 99	
HbA1c (%)			6.3		≥ 6.5	6.0 - 6.4	4.8 - 5.9	
25-hydroxy-Vitamin D (ng/mL)		12			≤ 14	15 - 29	30 - 100	
Uric Acid (mg/dL)			7.2		≥ 8	7.0 - 7.9	3.4 - 6.9	
TSH (µIU/mL)				0.79	< 0.27 or > 4.20		0.27 - 4.20	
Homocysteine (umol/L)								

The normal range for TSH is 0.5 to 5.0. Normally, the brain releases just enough TSH to maintain the right amount of thyroid hormones in the body. If the thyroid gland is not producing enough hormones, the brain releases more TSH to make the thyroid work harder to produce the hormones needed by the body to function normally.

Hypothyroidism occurs when the thyroid is underactive.

Hypothyroidism causes symptoms such as weight gain, tiredness, dry skin, constipation, a feeling of being too cold, and frequent irregular menstrual periods in women. More importantly, hypothyroidism increases your risk of heart disease for several reasons. First of all, it weakens the heart muscles. This means the heart cannot pump as vigorously as it should. As a result, the amount it ejects with every beat is reduced. If left untreated, this may lead to heart failure. In patients with stable heart failure, hypothyroidism can worsen the condition.

Furthermore, hypothyroidism promotes the oxidation of cholesterol, thereby increasing LDLs (bad cholesterol particles) circulating in the blood. It accelerates plaque buildup and development of coronary artery disease. Finally, hypothyroidism reduces the amount of nitric oxide in the endothelium (lining of the blood vessels), causing it to harden. Nitric oxide is the main chemical released by endothelial cells that maintains the health of blood vessels. Low levels of this substance results in endothelial dysfunction, which can lead to full-blown heart disease.

On the other hand, if there are too many thyroid hormones circulating in the body, the brain ceases to release TSH (leading to low TSH) which stops the thyroid from making more hormones. This condition wherein the thyroid is overactive is called **hyperthyroidism**. Hyperthyroidism causes symptoms such as weight loss, rapid heart rate, nervousness, irritability, diarrhea, a feeling of being too hot, and irregular menstrual periods for women.

Like hypothyroidism, it increases your risk of heart disease. In hyperthyroidism, the thyroid hormones increase both the force and rate of contraction of the heart. As a result, it makes the heart work harder than usual until it becomes exhausted. Although rare, heart failure can result from an untreated overactive thyroid. If there is an existing heart disease, hyperthyroidism can worsen the condition, making it very difficult to treat.

Underactive Thyroid	Overactive Thyroid
Makes you lose hair and gain weight. Raises your blood cholesterol, which increases your risk of heart disease.	Will drop your cholesterol level, but will also make you lose muscle and bone mass. It will also put you at high risk for abnormal rhythms called *atrial fibrillation*, which increases your risk for strokes.
The higher your TSH level, the higher your chances for developing heart disease.	
Thyroid hormone medication can easily correct this problem.	We need to find the cause of this problem in order to correct the condition.

Both hypothyroidism and hyperthyroidism can be very subtle in presentation. Often, they do not occur with the typical symptoms that doctors usually expect, so physicians often do not test you for these diseases. However, studies have shown that even the mildest form of thyroid disease can increase the risk of heart disease and worsen an existing heart condition. That is why it is important to include a thyroid function test on every heart disease prevention plan.

Your goal should be BETWEEN 0.27 TO 4.2.

25-hydroxy-Vitamin D

Laboratory Test	Notes	High Risk	Intermediate Risk	Optimal	High Risk Range	Intermediate Risk Range	Optimal Range	Previous Results
Insulin (µU/mL)				3	≥ 12	10 - 11	3 - 9	
Free Fatty Acid (mmol/L)		1.05			> 0.7	0.6 - 0.7	≤ 0.59	
Glucose (mg/dL)		286			≤ 55 or > 125	56-69 or 100-125	70 - 99	
HbA1c (%)			6.3		≥ 6.5	6.0 - 6.4	4.8 - 5.9	
25-hydroxy-Vitamin D (ng/mL)		12			≤ 14	15 - 29	30 - 100	
Uric Acid (mg/dL)			7.2		≥ 8	7.0 - 7.9	3.4 - 6.9	
TSH (µIU/mL)				0.79	< 0.27 or > 4.20		0.27 - 4.20	
Homocysteine (µmol/L)								

Low vitamin D levels put you at high risk for fractures, osteoporosis, bone loss, and coronary artery disease.

Several studies have shown that vitamin D deficiency increases the risk of heart disease and is linked to other well-known heart disease risk factors, such as high blood pressure, obesity, and diabetes. It also decreases your immunity and increases the incidence of cancers.

The best way to increase your vitamin D level is to expose your skin to sunlight every day for at least 10 to 15 minutes. If you can't stay out in the sun frequently, then you have to take vitamin D supplements.

Your vitamin D3 level should be checked regularly. If the level is low, no matter how much calcium you take in your diet, it will not be absorbed. You need normal or high levels of vitamin D for the absorption of calcium. Low calcium puts you at high risk for brittle bones and fractures.

Your goal should be MORE THAN 30.

Uric acid is a substance produced from the breakdown of proteins in the foods we eat.

Over time, too much uric acid in the blood can lead to the formation of needle-like crystals in the joints. These crystals trigger a condition more commonly known as **gout**. It is a form of arthritis characterized by sudden onset of severe swelling and tenderness of joints, usually in the big toe.

Laboratory Test	Notes	High Risk	Intermediate Risk	Optimal	High Risk Range	Intermediate Risk Range	Optimal Range	Previous Results
Insulin (µU/mL)				3	≥ 12	10 - 11	3 - 9	
Free Fatty Acid (mmol/L)		1.05			> 0.7	0.6 - 0.7	≤ 0.59	
Glucose (mg/dL)		286			≤ 55 or > 125	56-69 or 100-125	70 - 99	
HbA1c (%)			6.3		≥ 6.5	6.0 - 6.4	4.8 - 5.9	
25-hydroxy-Vitamin D (ng/mL)		12			≤ 14	15 - 29	30 - 100	
Uric Acid (mg/dL)			7.2		≥ 8	7.0 - 7.9	3.4 - 6.9	
TSH (µIU/mL)				0.79	< 0.27 or > 4.20		0.27 - 4.20	
Homocysteine (umol/L)								

Your goal should be LESS THAN 7.

A long time ago, uric acid level was used to diagnose gouty arthritis. Now, it is considered a potential risk factor for heart disease. Researchers have found that most people with heart disease (including those who died from it) had high levels of uric acid. In fact, the study showed that even those uric acid levels that are not high enough to cause gout can still lead to heart disease.

High uric acid levels are also found in other conditions such as hypertension, hyperlipidemia (high cholesterol, high triglycerides), obesity, and insulin resistance syndrome, which are all known risk factors for heart disease. This could explain why uric acid is associated with heart disease in the first place.

Checking for uric acid is important because it can indicate heart disease or other conditions that can cause heart disease. The higher the uric acid, the greater the risk.

What Increases Uric Acid Level?

Food

All organ meats, beef, chicken, gravies, bacon, sausages, game meats, anchovies, sardines, mackerel, scallops, herring, beans and lentils, oatmeal, wheat germ, wheat bran, peas, mushrooms, spinach, asparagus, cauliflower, breads (because of the yeast), corn syrup, fruits, and fructose (honey, agave nectar, high fructose corn syrup, and table sugar)

Drinks

Alcoholic beverages (particularly beer and wine), caffeinated beverages (teas, coffee, and sodas), and other beverages sweetened with corn syrup

Medicines

Aspirin, ascorbic acid, cisplatin, diazoxide, diuretics, epinephrine, ethambutol, levodopa, methyldopa, nicotinic acid, phenothiazines, and theophyline

RECOMMENDATION: Learn more about sugar, starch, and saturated fat and how to avoid them by reading the book *Eat This, Lose That* by Kota J. Reddy, M.D. (available at www.reddybread.com).

8

platelet and coagulation

More than 43 million people in the U.S. take aspirin every day. This drug helps prevent heart attacks and strokes by stopping the platelets from forming blood clots.

Laboratory Test	Notes	High Risk	Intermediate Risk	Optimal	High Risk Range	Intermediate Risk Range	Optimal Range	Previous Results 3/9/2011
Platelets AspirinWorks· (urine) (pg/mg of creatinine)				1000	> 1500		≤ 1500	

Aspirin does this by reducing the production of **thromboxane,** the chemical that makes platelets sticky and makes other substances in the blood adhere to them and form clots.

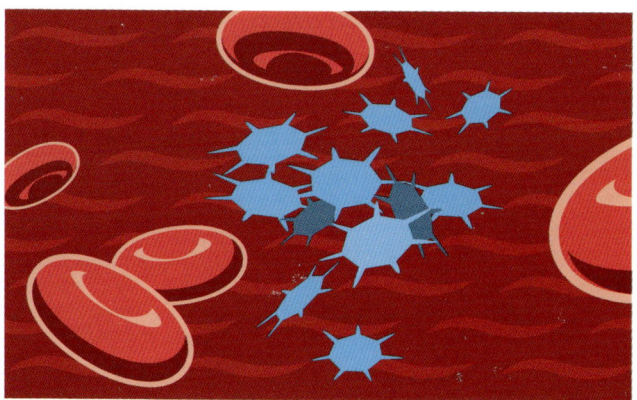

Platelets aggregating to form a clot inside an artery

However, research has demonstrated that up to 25% of these individuals may not benefit from the anti-clotting effect of aspirin and are three times more likely to die from a heart attack or stroke. This is why doctors are now beginning to recognize the importance of testing for aspirin effect.

With the AspirinWorks® test, you and your doctor can be sure your aspirin is working with a simple urine test that accurately determines aspirin effect by measuring levels of **11-dehydro thromboxane B2,** the chemical biomarker of thromboxane. A low level of the biomarker in the urine means that aspirin is working to reduce thromboxane production. High levels of the biomarker may mean that your dosage of aspirin is not effective for decreasing the risk of a heart attack or stroke, and it's time for you and your doctor to consider increasing the dose or changing your treatment strategy.

AspirinWorks® Flow Chart

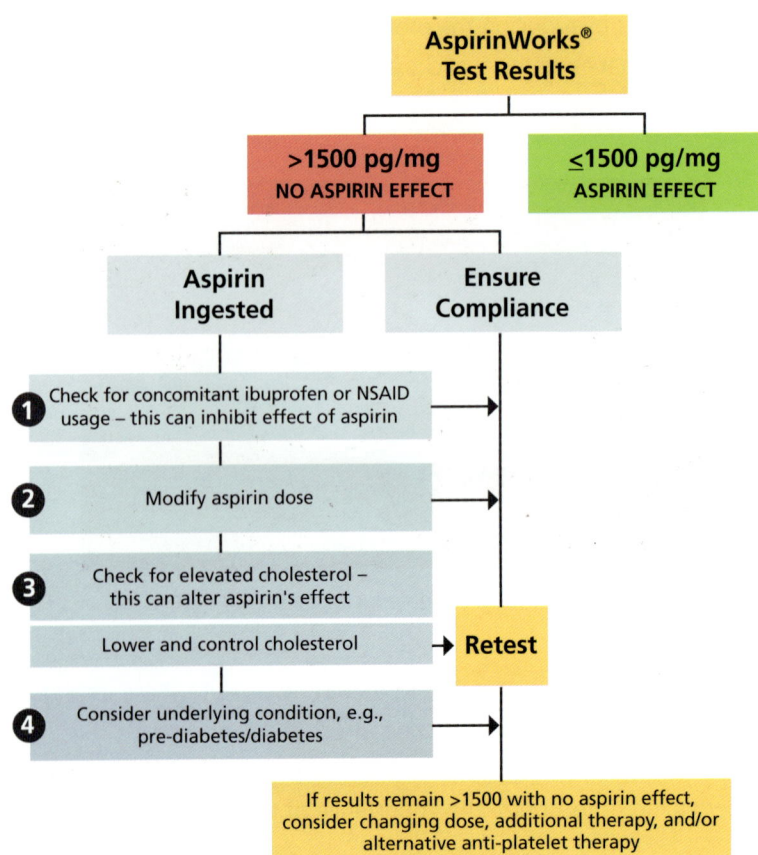

Plavix® is the brand name for clopidogrel and is the world's second best-selling drug. Like aspirin, Plavix® helps prevent heart attacks and strokes by inhibiting the function of platelets in forming blood clots.

Laboratory Test	Notes	High Risk	Intermediate Risk	Optimal	High Risk Range	Intermediate Risk Range	Optimal Range	Previous Results 3/9/2011
Platelet Genetics CYP2C19*				*1/*1		Estimated Genotype Frequency: *1/*1 (~60-70%), *1/*2 (~20-30%), *2/*2 (~2-3%), *1/*3 (<1%), *2/*3 (<0.05%), *3/*3 (<0.01%)		

However, patients with certain genetic variants (called *2 and *3) in the CYP2C19 gene may not receive the full benefit of clopidogrel. They poorly metabolize the drug into an active form and therefore are at an increased risk for forming blood clots. Another genetic variant (*17) enhances conversion of Plavix® into its active form. Patients with this variant, especially two copies, may be at increased risk of bleeding. The CYP2C19 test is a genetic test that can help doctors identify these patients and in time change treatment strategy. This test will report whether a patient is a poor, intermediate, or extensive metabolizer of Plavix®.

CYP2C19 variant(s)	Metabolizer type	Genotype
NONE present	EM – extensive "normal" metabolizer	*1/*1
ONE *2 or *3 present	IM – intermediate metabolizer	*1/*2, *1/*3
TWO *2 or *3 present	PM – poor metabolizer	*2/*2, *2/*3, *3/*3
ONE or TWO *17 present	UM – ultrarapid metabolizers	*1/*17, *17/*17
*17 plus EITHER *2 or *3	"unknown" metabolizer status	*2/*17, *3/*17

Laboratory Test	Notes	High Risk	Intermediate Risk	Optimal	High Risk Range	Intermediate Risk Range	Optimal Range	Previous Results 3/9/2011
Coagulation Genetics Factor V Leiden				Arg/Arg		Optimal=Non-carrier (Arg/Arg); At Risk=(Arg/Gln or Gln/Gln)		
Prothrombin Mutation				G/G		Optimal=Non-carrier (G/G); At Risk=(G/A or A/A)		

Factor V Leiden is the name of a specific gene mutation that results in an increased risk of developing a type of blood clot called a deep venous thrombosis (DVT).

People carrying the Factor V Leiden mutation have a five times greater risk of developing thrombosis than the rest of the population.

The prothrombin mutation is also a gene mutation in which affected individuals produce too much prothrombin protein. The prothrombin protein, also called Factor II, is a protein that helps blood to clot. A surplus of this protein is dangerous because, like Factor V Leiden, it can cause deep venous thrombosis.

DVTs occur most often in the legs, although they can also occur in other parts of the body, including the brain, eyes, liver, and kidneys. Factor V Leiden also increases the risk that clots will break away from their original site and travel through the bloodstream. These clots can lodge in the lungs, where they are known as pulmonary emboli, and can be fatal. The risk is increased in situations such as pregnancy, oral contraceptive use, estrogen therapy, malignancy, diabetes mellitus, immobilization, or surgery.

These tests determine presence or absence of the mutations. It gives doctors the ability to detect those patients who are at risk and the opportunity to prevent venous thrombosis through special management.

Factor V Leiden

Genotype	Result
Arg/Arg	Non-carrier (no risk)
Arg/Gln	Carrier (3 to 8 times more risk)
Gln/Gln	Carrier (10 to 100 times more risk)

Prothrombin Mutation

Genotype	Result
G/G	Non-carrier (no risk)
G/A	Carrier (3 to 8 times more risk)
A/A	Carrier (> 10 times more risk)

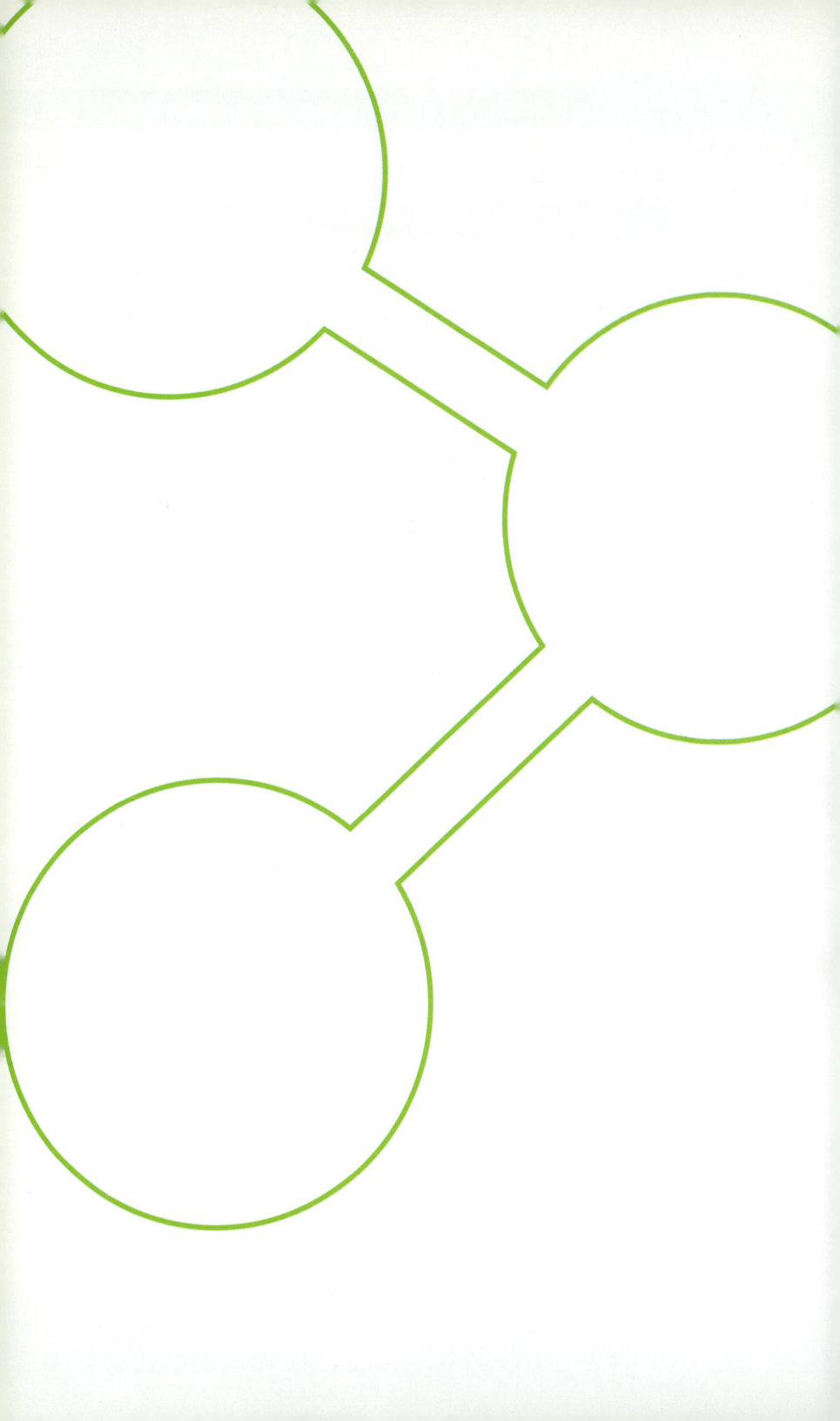

9

newly added tests to estimate your risk

Galectin-3 is a protein that binds to a certain class of carbohydrates during episodes of injury and inflammation to promote fibrogenesis (scarring).

	Laboratory Test	Notes	High Risk	Intermediate Risk	Optimal	High Risk Range	Intermediate Risk Range	Optimal Range	Previous Results
Myocardial Stress	NT-proBNP (pg/mL)			323		> 449	125 - 449	< 125	
	Galectin-3 (ng/mL)		27.2			> 25.9	17.9 - 25.9	< 17.9	

In people who have had a heart attack or have chronic high blood pressure, an elevated galectin-3 level may causes changes in the heart structure, such as thickening and stiffening of the heart muscle, thus increasing the risk for developing heart failure.

Galectin-3

Galectin-3	Risk
<17.8 ng/mL	Low risk
17.8 to 25.9 ng/mL	Intermediate risk (2x higher risk of hospitalization or death from cardiovascular causes)
>25.9 ng/mL	High risk (3x higher risk of hospitalization or death from cardiovascular causes)

This test allows identification of high levels before the onset of heart abnormalities. If identified early, galectin-3 protein activity can be blocked using drugs or natural inhibitors found in vegetables.

Eat more vegetables and stay away from sugars and starches.

Role of galectin-3 in Heart Failure

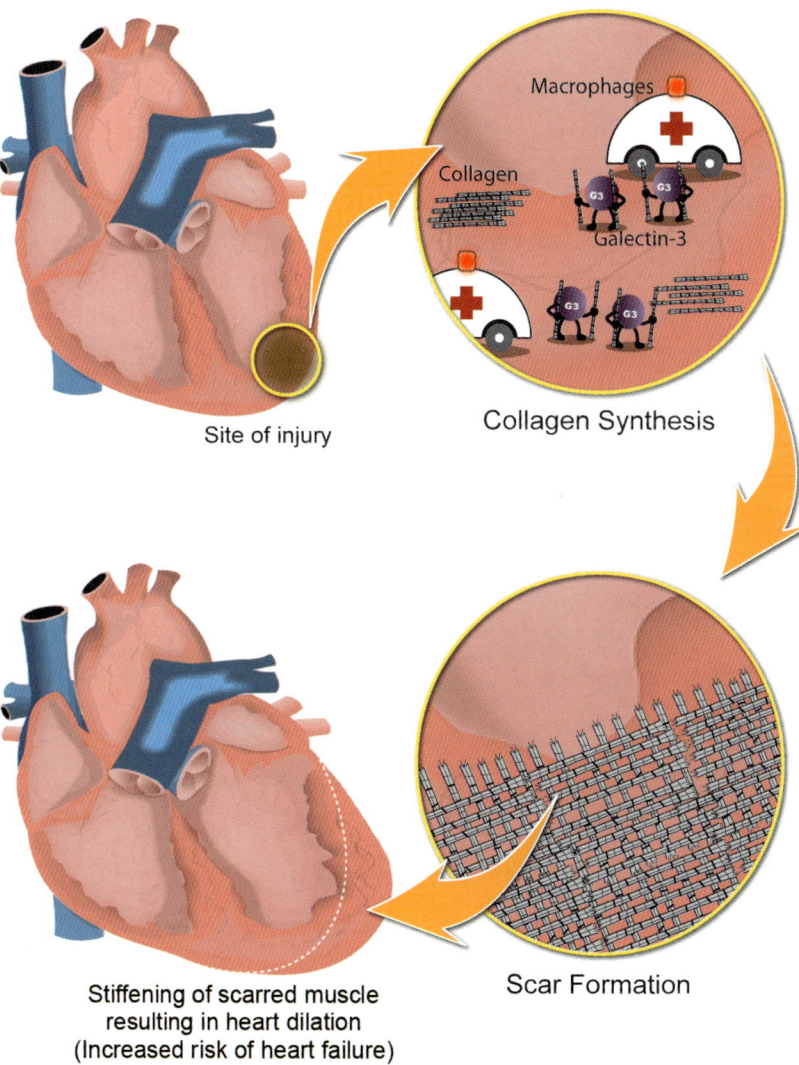

Site of injury

Collagen Synthesis

Scar Formation

Stiffening of scarred muscle
resulting in heart dilation
(Increased risk of heart failure)

Your goal should be LESS THAN 17.8.

Plant sterols and stanols are substances that occur naturally in small amounts in many grains, vegetables, fruits, legumes, nuts, and seeds.

They serve no human purpose and under normal circumstances are not absorbed by the body. However, people vary in their cholesterol balance — the amount they produce or synthesize, absorb, and excrete. Due to genetic differences, some people (hyperabsorbers) may absorb plant sterols and stanols. Therefore, we can use the concentrations of plant sterols and stanols in the blood as clinical markers of cholesterol absorption. Several large clinical studies have shown that elevated plasma noncholesterol sterols are a powerful indicator of heart disease risk.

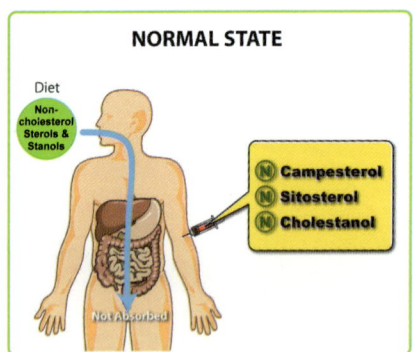
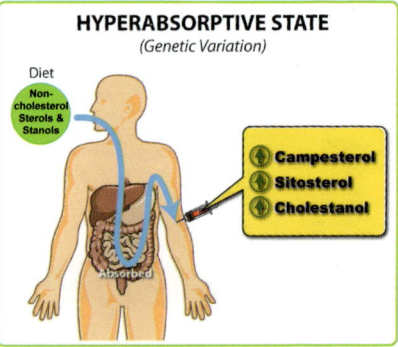

This test measures three noncholesterol sterols as well as a stanol:

- **Beta-sitosterol**, **campesterol** and **cholestanol** serve as markers of cholesterol absorption.

- **Desmosterol** serves as a marker of cholesterol synthesis.

Reference Range

Absorption Marker	State		
	Hyper-Absorption	Normal	Hypo-Absorption
Campesterol (ug/mL)	>4.43	2.11 to 4.43	<2.11
Campesterol Ratio (10² mmol/mol Cholesterol)	>240	115–240	<115
Sitosterol (ug/mL)	>3.17	1.43 to 3.17	<1.43
Sitosterol Ratio (10² mmol/mol Cholesterol)	>168	76–168	<76
Cholestanol (ug/mL)	>3.47	2.02 to 3.47	<2.02
Cholestanol Ratio (10² mmol/mol Cholesterol)	>194	117–194	<117

Synthesis Marker	State		
	Hyper-Synthesis	Normal	Hypo-Synthesis
Desmosterol (ug/mL)	≥1.28	0.50 to 1.27	≤0.49
Desmosterol Ratio (10² mmol/mol Cholesterol)	≥65	31–64	≤31

Testing for plasma sterol levels will provide information on whether a patient is more of an absorber, a synthesizer, both or neither. It will help physicians personalize drug therapy and more effectively manage lipid levels.

Fatty acids are important constituents of cell membranes in our body, and having the correct composition is vital to our cardiovascular and overall health.

Laboratory Test	Notes	High Risk	Intermediate Risk	Optimal	High Risk Range	Intermediate Risk Range	Optimal Range	Previous Results
Index HS-Omega-3 Index® (RBC EPA+DHA)ᵃ		3.0			< 4.0%	4.0% - 8.0%	> 8.0%	

Comments:

Your HS-Omega-3 Index is well below the target range of 8%.

The HS-Omega-3 Index is the EPA+DHA content of RBC membranes. Increasing the intake of EPA+DHA by 1 to 2 grams (1,000 - 2,000 mg) per day, from either oily fish or fish oil supplements, should significantly improve the index. The exact amount of EPA+DHA needed will vary person to person. A re-check should be done in 3 - 4 months.

Omega-3 Fatty Acids			
Fatty Acids	Range	Current	Previous
Omega-3 Total	0.1% - 14.1%	5.9%	
Alpha-Linolenic (ALA)	0.1% - 0.4%	0.2%	
Docosapentaenoic (DPA)	0.6% - 4.1%	2.8%	
Eicosapentaenoic (EPA)	0.1% - 2.5%	0.5%	
Docosahexaenoic (DHA)	0.1% - 8.4%	2.5%	

Omega-6 Fatty Acids			
Fatty Acids	Range	Current	Previous
Omega-6 Total	28.6% - 44.5%	35.6%	
Arachidonic (AA)	10.5% - 23.3%	16.6%	
Linoleic (LA)	4.6% - 21.3%	10.3%	

Other Fatty Acids			
Fatty Acids	Range	Current	Previous
cis-Monounsaturated Total	11.5% - 20.5%	17.3%	
Saturated Total	36.6% - 42.0%	40.9%	
Trans Total	<0.1% - 1.8%	1.6%	

The two fatty acids essential for health are omega-3 and omega-6. These are essential because they cannot be manufactured by the body and must come from food. Omega-3 fatty acids are needed for brain and eye development of the growing fetus during pregnancy and for maintaining and promoting health throughout life. They also have beneficial effects on cardiovascular risk. Omega-6 fatty acids play an important role in brain and heart function, and in normal growth and development.

	Common Forms	Common Sources
Omega-3 fatty acid	Eicosapentaenoic (EPA) Docosahexaenoic (DHA) Alpha linolenic acids (ALA)	**EPA and DHA:** fatty fish such as salmon, white tuna, mackerel, rainbow trout, herring, halibut, and sardines **ALA:** canola or soybean oil, walnuts, and ground flaxseed or flaxseed oil
Omega-6 fatty acid	Linoleic acid (LA)	Vegetable oils (e.g., corn, sunflower, safflower, and soy), salad dressing, nuts, whole wheat bread, and chicken

This test measures the fatty acid profile of the red blood cell membranes and reports The HS Omega-3 Index® to assess the risk for heart disease. This risk can be reduced by taking fish oil supplements and by reducing saturated and trans fats in the diet.

Reference Range

HS-Omega-3 Index	Relative Risk	Treatment Options
< 4%	High risk 10x increased risk for sudden cardiac death	1-2 g/day of EPA+DHA from oily fish and/or fish oil supplements
4 – 8%	Intermediate risk	0.5-1 g/day of EPA+DHA from oily fish and/or fish oil supplements
> 8%	Optimal	

Your goal should be MORE THAN 8%.

Vitamin B$_{12}$ is essential in making blood cells and maintaining a healthy nervous system.

Laboratory Test	Notes	High Risk	Intermediate Risk	Optimal	High Risk Range	Intermediate Risk Range	Optimal Range	Previous Results
Insulin (µU/mL)		47			≥ 12	10 - 11	3 - 9	
Free Fatty Acid (mmol/L)		0.86			> 0.7	0.6 - 0.7	≤ 0.59	
Glucose (mg/dL)					≤ 55 or > 125	56-69 or 100-125	70 - 99	
HbA1c (%)					≥ 6.5	5.7 - 6.4	≤ 5.6	
25-hydroxy-Vitamin D (ng/mL)		6			≤ 14	15 - 29	30 - 100	
Homocysteine (µmol/L)				10	> 13	11 - 13	≤ 10	
Vitamin B$_{12}$ (pg/mL)				675	< 211	211 - 299	≥ 300	

It is estimated that 5% to 40% of the elderly population have vitamin B$_{12}$ deficiency due to reduced absorption. This increases the risk for pernicious anemia, cancer, nervous system disorders, and cardiovascular disease.

This test will assess your risk and provide your doctor with information to customize your treatment plan. Once the diagnosis of vitamin B$_{12}$ deficiency has been confirmed, efficient treatment can be ensured either by injections every two to three months or by a daily dose of 1 mg of vitamin B$_{12}$. Vitamin B$_{12}$ administration will increase red blood cell production, which may increase the need for iron supplementation as well.

Reference Range

	High Risk Range	Intermediate Risk Range	Optimal Range
Vitamin B$_{12}$ (pg/mL)	>946 and < 211	211 - 299	300 - 946

Folic acid is a water-soluble B vitamin, derived solely from food, such as egg yolks, beef, poultry, and fish. Many people, especially the elderly, are deficient in this important nutrient.

Inadequate levels of folate increase the risk for heart disease and stroke.

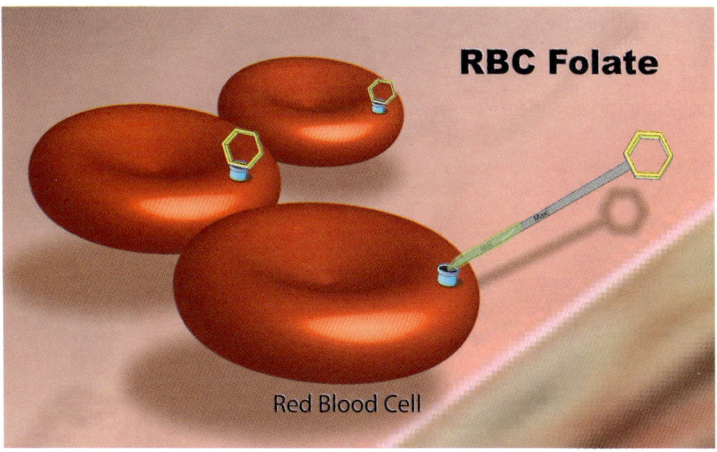

RBC Folate

Red Blood Cell

This test will measure the amount of folate inside the red blood cells (RBCs), which is an accurate reflection of the body's folate status and supply. If your level is low, your doctor may suggest folic acid supplements to improve your overall health.

Reference Range

	High Risk Range	Intermediate Risk Range	Optimal Range
RBC Folate (ng/mL)	≤ 467		≥ 468

Cystatin C is a test that determines kidney function.

Laboratory Test	Notes	High Risk	Intermediate Risk	Optimal	High Risk Range	Intermediate Risk Range	Optimal Range	Previous Results
Renal Cystatin C (mg/L)				0.86	≥ 1.04	0.96 - 1.03	≤ 0.95	

It is used as a substitute for eGFR (estimated Glomerular Filtration Rate), a measure of how well the kidneys filter waste products from the blood. High levels of cystatin C may indicate an acute or chronic kidney dysfunction. Studies have also shown that cystatin C levels can predict new-onset or deteriorating cardiovascular disease.

Several causative factors linked to high cystatin C levels have been identified such as smoking, obesity, liver disease, diabetes, and heart disease.

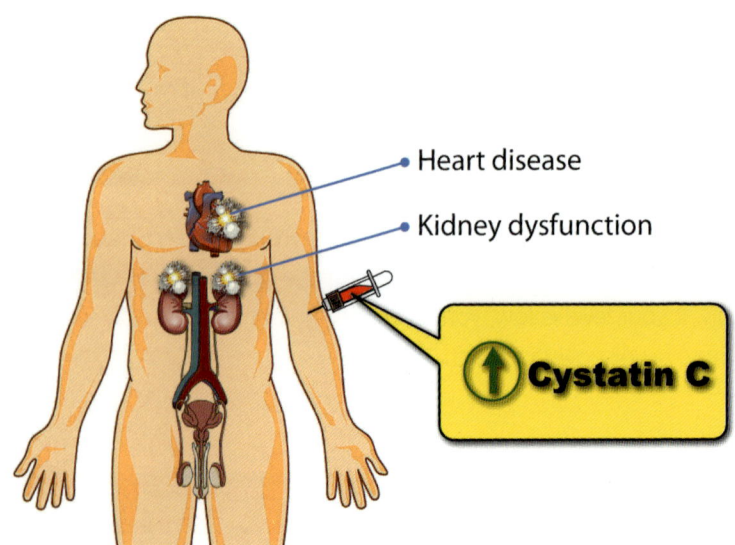

Heart disease

Kidney dysfunction

Cystatin C

Your goal should be LESS THAN 1.04.

People at risk for blood clots are often prescribed the blood thinner warfarin. However, the dose of warfarin required to achieve a stable therapeutic effect varies widely among individuals.

The consequences of incorrect dosage are severe and, in some cases, life-threatening. If too little warfarin is prescribed, the threat of blood clots will remain. But if too much drug is given, uncontrolled bleeding can result. Although a variety of factors influence a patient's ideal dose of warfarin, the genetic variations in the CYP2C9 and VKORC1 genes play an important part. Changes in the CYP2C9 and VKORC1 genes can affect how you respond to warfarin. Warfarin response testing looks for common variants in these two genes. The test is run on cells taken from a cheek swab or a blood sample.

People have two copies of each of these genes, one from each parent. This test tells you what combination of CYP2C9 and VKORC1 genes you have. It is possible to have zero, one, or two gene variants for each gene. If testing finds one or more gene variants, the results are reliable.

CYP2C9 and VKORC1 Genes

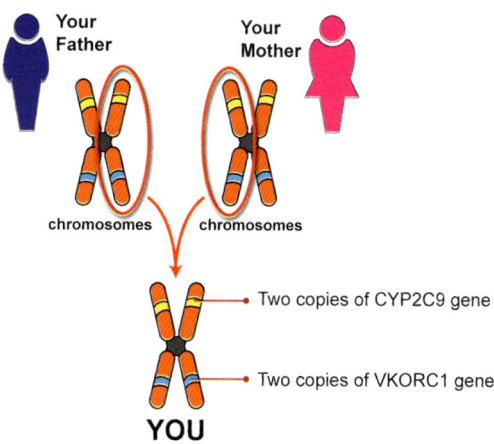

Your Father

Your Mother

chromosomes   chromosomes

Two copies of CYP2C9 gene

Two copies of VKORC1 gene

YOU

- The "normal" form of the CYP2C9 gene is called *1. Testing usually looks for the two most common variants in the CYP2C9 gene called *2 and *3. These variants are more common in people with European ancestry. Some tests also look for additional variants that are more common in African American people.

- A single VKORC1 gene variant, called -1639G>A, explains most warfarin response problems from this gene. People with one or more copies of the "A" variant are more sensitive to warfarin than those with "G" variants.

CYP2C9	Status	Warfarin Dose
No variant	Normal metabolizer	Follow current guidelines for warfarin therapy
One variant	Intermediate metabolizer	Reduce the dose For *2 ~17% lower For *3 ~37% lower
Two variants	Poor metabolizer	Reduce the dose further

VKORC1	Status	Warfarin Dose
No A variant	Low sensitivity	Increase the dose
One A variant	Intermediate sensitivity (considered normal)	Follow the current guidelines for warfarin therapy
Two A variants	High sensitivity	Reduce the dose further

The Warfarin Sensitivity test determines how a patient's genotype responds to warfarin. Patients who have variations in the CYP2C9 genes are said to metabolize warfarin more slowly than usual, thus requiring a lower than average warfarin dose, especially during the first weeks of treatment. Patients with the A variants at position -1639 of the VKORC1 gene are more sensitive to warfarin than those without variants and would also require a lower dose of warfarin. If you need to take or are taking warfarin, having this test will aid physicians in administering the optimal warfarin dose and potentially reduce the risk of adverse events.

The MTHFR gene provides instructions for making an enzyme called methylenetetrahydrofolate reductase.

Laboratory Test	Notes	High Risk	Intermediate Risk	Optimal	High Risk Range	Intermediate Risk Range	Optimal Range	Previous Results
Coagulation Genetics Factor V Leiden*				Arg/Arg	Optimal=Non-carrier (Arg/Arg); At Risk=(Arg/Gln or Gln/Gln)			
Prothrombin Mutation*				G/G	Optimal=Non-carrier (G/G); At Risk=(G/A or A/A)			
MTHFR* (Methylenetetrahydrofolate Reductase)			T/T		Estimated Genotype Frequency: C/C (~49.3%), C/T (~39.8%), T/T (~10.9%)			

This enzyme is important for a chemical reaction involving forms of the B-vitamin folate (also called folic acid). Specifically, this enzyme is needed in the conversion of the amino acid homocysteine to another amino acid, methionine. The body uses methionine to make proteins and other important compounds.

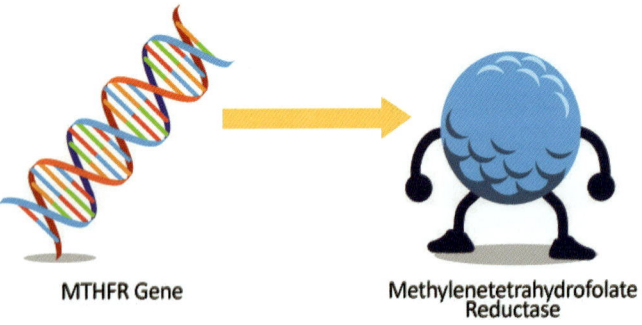

MTHFR Gene   Methylenetetrahydrofolate Reductase

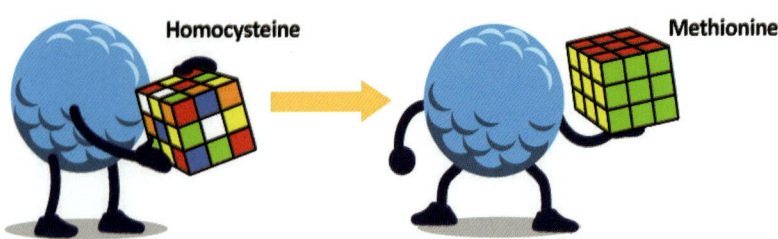

Homocysteine   Methionine

This test identifies mutations in the MTHFR gene. Mutations in the gene impair the function of methylenetetrahydrofolate reductase enzyme in converting homocysteine to methionine. As a result, homocysteine builds up in the bloodstream and in turn increases your risk for heart disease and stroke. Individuals with the MTHFR gene variant may also have a higher blood pressure.

MTHFR	Status	Relative Risk	Warfarin Dose
No variant	Normal homocysteine level	None	Maintain adequate vitamin B and folate status
One variant	↑ homocysteine level	↑ CVD risk when folate status or dietary folate is low	↑ Vitamin B supplementation (Folate, B_{12}, B_6)
Two variants	↑↑ homocysteine level	↑↑ CVD risk when folate status or dietary folate is low	↑↑ Vitamin B supplementation (Folate, B_{12}, B_6, B_2)

If you have the variant MTHFR gene, your physician may give you high levels of vitamin B_{12} and folate supplements in order to prevent serum homocysteine concentration from becoming elevated. Also, eating more vegetables increases your methionine level.

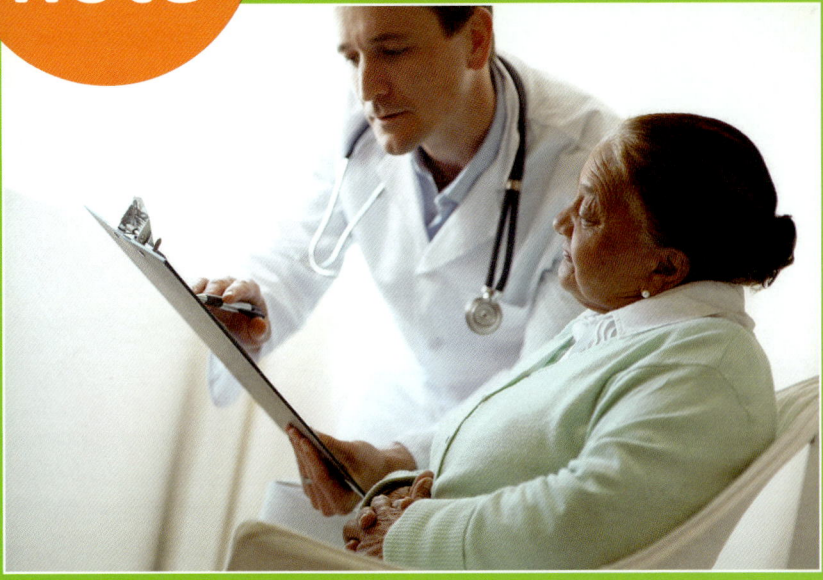

Thank you for taking time to learn how to interpret your advance cardiovascular profile report from Health Diagnostic Laboratory, Inc. The next step is to talk to your doctor to find out if you are at risk and what you can do to improve your health.

Start learning about diet, especially about sugar, starch, and saturated fat and how to avoid them. Maintain regular follow-ups with your primary care doctor and take your medications (when necessary) as prescribed.

Remember, sticking with a regular testing regimen is critical to your path to better health. It allows your doctor to monitor the effects of medication and treatment. With periodic monitoring of your results, a personal treatment plan can be fine-tuned for improving your total health. Your plan may include medication, diet, and lifestyle recommendations and, in many cases, you can halt or even reverse the progression of disease.

Criteria to Check for Metabolic Syndrome*

○ **Central obesity**
Waist circumference: ≥ 102cm or 40 inches (male)
                                    ≥ 88cm or 36 inches (female)
BMI more than 30m^2/kg

○ **Triglycerides** greater than 150mg/dl

○ **HDL** <40mg/dl (male); <50mg/dl (female)

○ **Blood pressure** ≥ 130/85mmHg

○ **Fasting blood glucose level** ≥ 110mg/dl

○ Presence of **small LDL particles**

*Three or more of the above is required to diagnose Metabolic Syndrome.

Criteria to Check for Insulin Resistance

○ **Triglycerides/HDL Ratio** greater than 3.5
*shows insulin resistance and means that you
are at high risk for developing diabetes*

○ **HOMA-IR=Fasting Insulin x Fasting Glucose ÷ 22.5**
(Homeostasis Model Assessment of Insulin Resistance)
HOMA-IR more than 3.5 shows insulin resistance

Treatment Options for Abnormal Test Results

Test	Treatment
LDL-C	Lifestyle changes, statins
HDL-C	Lifestyle changes, niacin, statins, fibrates
LDL-P	Lifestyle changes, statins
sdLDL	Lifestyle changes, niacin (N), fibrates (F), statins (S), combination therapy (N+F+S)
Lp(a) mass	Niacin
Lp(a) cholesterol	Niacin
ApoB	Lifestyle changes, statins
ApoA-1	Statins, niacin
HDL2	Fish oil (FO), niacin, fibrates (F), combination therapy (FO+N+F)
ApoB/ApoA-1 ratio	Weight loss, lifestyle changes, statins, fibrates
FRP & Fibrinogen	Lifestyle changes, statins, fibrates, niacin, fish oil
Lp-PLA$_2$	Lifestyle changes, statins, fibrates, niacin
Myeloperoxidase (MPO)	Statins, niacin
NT-proBNP	Statins, lifestyle changes
Insulin & Glucose	Lifestyle changes, medication(s) for diabetes, fibrates
HbA1c	Dietary modification, lifestyle changes, medication(s) for diabetes
Free Fatty Acid	Lifestyle changes, niacin, fibrates
TSH	Thyroid hormone therapy
25-Hydroxy Vitamin D	Vitamin D supplements, fish like wild salmon, egg yolk
ApoE	Dietary modifications, lifestyle changes, fish oil
Triglycerides	Dietary modifications (low-fat diet)
HDL-P	Dietary modifications, niacin

NAME_____

DATE_____

Summary of My Advanced Cardiovascular Profile

TOTAL CHOLESTEROL

What is my total cholesterol? _____

Total Cholesterol = HDL + LDL + Triglycerides

Is my total cholesterol high? ○ yes ○ no

If your total cholesterol is high, you are eating a lot **sugar, starch,** and **saturated fat.**

NOTE: Cholesterol in the diet will not raise your total cholesterol significantly. It is the saturated fat in the diet that will increase your total cholesterol significantly.

LDL-C

Is my bad cholesterol high? ○ yes ○ no

If your bad cholesterol is high, you are eating a lot of **sugars, starches,** and **bad fats (saturated fat and trans fat).**

HDL-C

Is my good cholesterol low? ○ yes ○ no

If your good cholesterol is low, you are eating a lot of **sugar and starch.**

TRIGLYCERIDES

Are the fats in my blood high? ○ yes ○ no

If your triglycerides are high, you are eating a lot of **sugar and starch.**

NON-HDL CHOLESTEROL

What is my non-HDL cholesterol? _____

Non-HDL = Total cholesterol – HDL

Is my non-HDL cholesterol high? ○ yes ○ no

If your non-HDL cholesterol is high, you are eating a lot of **sugar and starch.**

APOB

Is my apoB high? ○ ○
yes no

ApoB is the "key" that lets the bad cholesterol enter the artery wall to form plaque. If your apoB is high, you are eating a lot of **sugar** and **starch.**

LDL-P

Do I have a lot of LDL particles in my blood? ○ ○
yes no

LDL-P is the number of particles carrying the cholesterol and triglycerides in the blood. The higher the number, the more plaque can buildup in the arteries. If your LDL-P is high, you are eating a lot of **sugar** and **starch.**

sdLDL

Are my LDL particles small in size? ○ ○
yes no

Small LDL particles build plaque in the arteries faster because they stay in the blood longer and can penetrate the artery wall easily. If your LDL particles are small in size, you are eating a lot of **sugar and starch.**

APOA-1

Is the protein that makes my good cholesterol low? ○ ○
yes no

If your apoA-1 is low, you are eating a lot of **sugar and starch.**

HDL-P

Do I have a lot of HDL particles in my blood? ○ ○
yes no

HDL-P is the number of particles carrying the good cholesterol in the blood. The higher the number, the cleaner your arteries are. If your HDL-P is low, you are eating a lot of **sugar and starch.**

HDL2

Are my HDL particles large in size? ○ ○
yes no

The larger the HDL particles, the better. They clean the arteries faster and accelerate the reversal of heart disease. The HDL particles decrease in size when you eat a lot of **sugar and starch.**

APOB/APOA-1 RATIO

Is my apoB/apoA-1 ratio high?   ◯ yes ◯ no

If your apoB/apoA-1 ratio is high, you are at high risk for plaque formation and heart disease. Eating a lot of **sugar** and **starch** increases your apoB and lowers your apoA-1, thus increasing this ratio.

LP(a) MASS

Are my "deadly cholesterol" particles large in size?   ◯ yes ◯ no

Lp(a) is an additional protein attached to the bad cholesterol that increases your risk for plaque and blood clot formation, thus increasing your chances for heart attack and stroke.

LP(a) CHOLESTEROL

Is my Lp(a) cholesterol high?   ◯ yes ◯ no

If your Lp(a) cholesterol is high, you are at high risk for forming plaque and blood clots, thus increasing your chances for heart attack and stroke.

Can you have "high" Lp(a) mass and "normal" Lp(a) cholesterol?   ◯ yes ◯ no

Is it dangerous?   ◯ yes ◯ no

Can you have "high" Lp(a) mass and "high" Lp(a) cholesterol?   ◯ yes ◯ no

Is it dangerous?   ◯ yes ◯ no

CRP

Is there inflammation in my body?   ◯ yes ◯ no

CRP level is high if there is inflammation occurring in the body, including the coronary arteries, which increases your risk for heart attack. However, this is not specific because high CRP level can also occur if you have a lot of belly fat and during times of acute infection.

FIBRINOGEN

Is my fibrinogen high? ○ ○
                                            yes no

Fibrinogen is a fibrous protein that thickens the blood and promotes clotting. High levels will raise your risk for heart attack and stroke. If your fibrinogen level is high, you are eating a lot of **sugar, starch, and saturated fat.** High levels can also be seen with cigarette smoking, inactivity, old age, diabetes, and metabolic syndrome.

LP-PLA₂

Is there inflammation in my arteries? ○ ○
yes no

Lp-PLA₂ is specific for inflammation in the arteries. A high level signifies that there is a plaque somewhere getting ready to crack and cause a heart attack or stroke. If your Lp-PLA₂ level is high, you are eating a lot of **sugar, starch,** and **saturated fat.**

MPO

Is my myeloperoxidase level high? ○ ○
yes no

Myeloperoxidase is a substance that damages the endothelium (the inner lining of blood vessels) and promotes plaque formation and heart disease. If your MPO level is high, you are eating a lot of **sugar, starch, and saturated fat.**

NT-PROBNP

Is there stress or strain on my heart? ○ ○
yes no

A high level of NT-proBNP is a warning sign that the heart is continuously being stressed or strained. Conditions like congestive heart failure, atrial fibrillation, pulmonary hypertension, and sleep apnea can raise this level and put you at risk for heart attack and stroke.

ASPIRINWORKS

Will I benefit from aspirin? ○ ○
yes no

Aspirin therapy has been reported to reduce heart attack and stroke from 15% to 40%. This test will tell you if you will benefit from aspirin so that your physician can either increase your current dose or switch you to a more appropriate drug.

HBA1C		
Is my hemoglobin A1c high?	○ yes ○ no	This test determines how much your blood glucose has been controlled for the last three to four months. If this level is high, you probably have diabetes or your diabetes is uncontrolled and you are eating a lot of **sugar** and **starch.**
FREE FATTY ACID		
Do I have a lot of free fatty acids in my blood?	○ yes ○ no	If this level is high, you have insulin resistance or metabolic syndrome, which increases your risk for developing diabetes, and you have been eating a lot of **sugar** and **starch.**
VITAMIN D		
Is my vitamin D level normal?	○ yes ○ no	If your vitamin D is low, your risk of fracture, osteoporosis, bone loss, and coronary heart disease increases. You need exposure to sunlight at least 10 to 15 minutes a day plus vitamin D supplements.
TSH		
Is my thyroid normal?	○ yes ○ no	○ hypothyroid ○ hyperthyroid Abnormal thyroid function increases your risk of heart disease.
FACTOR V LEIDEN		
Do I carry the Factor V Leiden mutation?	○ yes ○ no	People carrying the Factor V Leiden gene mutation have a much greater risk of developing a type of blood clot called a deep venous thrombosis (DVT) than the rest of the population.
PROTHROMBIN MUTATION		
Is there a mutation in my prothrombin?	○ yes ○ no	A mutation in prothrombin increases your risk for blood clots especially in your veins. Talk to your doctor as you may need to be on blood thinner. Regular exercise, losing weight, quitting smoking, avoiding prolonged sitting or immobility may help lower this level.

What type of food should I avoid?   ○ sugar   ○ starch   ○ saturated fat

RECOMMENDATION: Learn more about sugar, starch, and saturated fat and how to avoid them by reading the book *Eat This, Lose That* by Kota J. Reddy, M.D. (available at www.reddybread.com).

GALECTIN-3

Is my galectin-3 high?   ○ ○
                               yes no

Galectin-3 is a protein that promotes scarring in the heart muscles causing the heart to be stiff, which increases your risk of heart failure. It can be blocked by using drugs or natural inhibitors found in vegetables.

NONCHOLESTEROL STEROLS/STANOLS

Am I absorbing cholesterol more than usual?   ○ ○
                               yes no

Am I producing cholesterol more than usual?   ○ ○
                               yes no

People vary in their cholesterol balance — the amounts they produce or synthesize, absorb, and excrete. Due to genetic differences, some people may absorb or synthesize cholesterol more than others. This test will provide information on whether a patient is more of an absorber, a synthesizer, both or neither. It will help physicians personalize drug therapy and more effectively manage lipid levels.

OMEGA-3 AND OMEGA-6 FATTY ACID PROFILE

Are my omega-3 and omega-6 fatty acid levels normal?   ○ ○
                               yes no

This test measures the fatty acid profile of the red blood cell membranes and reports The HS® Omega-3 Index to assess the risk for heart disease. This risk can be reduced by taking fish oil supplements and by reducing saturated and trans fats in the diet.

VITAMIN B_{12}

Is my vitamin B_{12} level normal?   ○ ○
                               yes no

Low vitamin B_{12} increases the risk for pernicious anemia, cancer, nervous system disorders, and cardiovascular disease. This test will assess your risk and provide your doctor with information to customize your treatment plan.

RBC FOLATE

Is my folic acid level normal?   ○ ○
                               yes no

Inadequate levels of folate increases the risk for heart disease and stroke. This test will measure the amount of folate inside the red blood cell, which is an accurate reflection of the body's folate status and supply. If your level is low, your doctor may suggest folic acid supplements to improve your overall health.

CYSTATIN C			
Do I have kidney dysfunction that I don't know about?	◯ yes	◯ no	High levels of cystatin C may indicate an acute or chronic kidney dysfunction, which can predict new-onset or deteriorating cardiovascular disease.

WARFARIN SENSITIVITY			
Do I metabolize warfarin more slowly than ususal?	◯ yes	◯ no	This test determines how a patient's genotype responds to warfarin. If you need to take or are taking warfarin, having this test will aid physicians in administering the optimal warfarin dose and potentially reduce the risk of adverse events.
Am I sensitive to warfarin's therapeutic effect?	◯ yes	◯ no	

METHYLENETETRAHYDROFOLATE REDUCTASE (MTHFR)			
Do I have a variant MTHFR gene?	◯ yes	◯ no	This test identifies mutations in the MTHFR gene. Mutations in the gene impair the function of methylenetetrahydrofolate reductase enzyme in converting homocysteine to methionine. As a result, homocysteine builds up in the bloodstream and in turn increases your risk for heart disease and stroke. Vitamin B_{12} and folate supplements may prevent homocysteine levels from becoming elevated.

What to eat when you want to get off your medications

Introducing: The "Reddy Bread"

An alternative to conventional bread which is both heart-healthy and diabetes-friendly, this product contains all-natural ingredients. They are blended with the nutritious combination of protein from soy and omega-3 from flax, which makes them healthier alternatives to white and wheat breads. Their low-carbohydrate nature and ability to maintain normal blood sugar make them an excellent choice for people who want to lose weight and for people who are battling diabetes.

The addiction to sugar and starch is no different from alcoholism, smoking, or cocaine abuse. In a recent study, rats were given a choice between sugar water and cocaine, and 94% of them chose sugar. Even rats that had previously been addicted to cocaine switched to sugar once it was a choice.

If you treat food like medication and eat non-addicting foods, you will never have to worry about your health.

Reddy Bread vs. Corn Tortilla: Effect on Blood Sugar Level

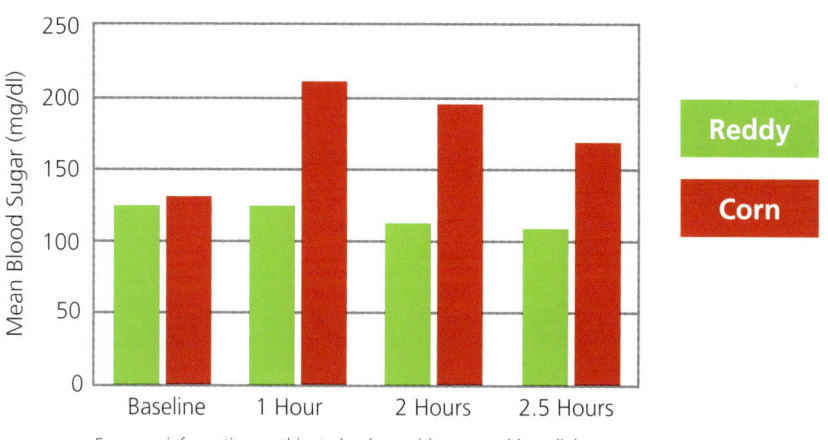

For more information on this study, please visit www.reddycardiology.com

Why is "Reddy Bread" good for diabetic patients?

A study was done to determine the effect of Reddy Bread on blood sugar levels of diabetic patients. Using a tortilla made with the same ingredients as this bread, the study showed that there was no increase in blood sugar, triglyceride, and cholesterol levels of diabetic patients at 1, 2, and 2.5 hours after eating the tortilla.

Eat This, Lose That! by Dr. Kota J. Reddy

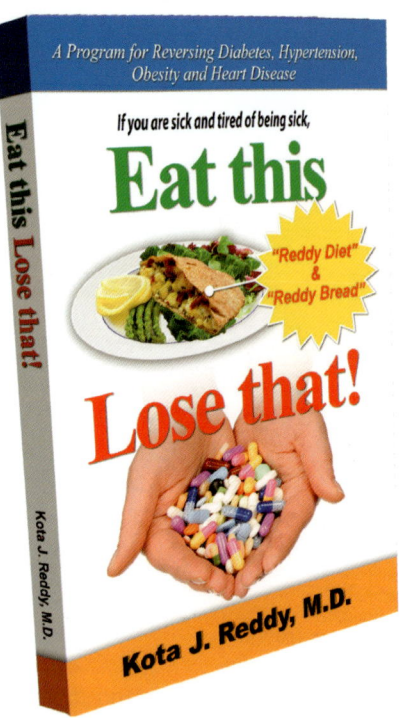

This book will help you:

- Reduce the number or eliminate the need of medications for your diabetes and high blood pressure
- Lose weight
- Improve your cholesterol levels

It will teach you how to eat the right foods without having to worry about:

- Counting calories
- The number of times you have to eat
- How much cholesterol you consume
- The amount of food you have to eat

Available at:
Reddy Cardiac Wellness
3519 Town Center Blvd. S. Suite A
Sugar Land, TX, 77479

www.reddybread.com

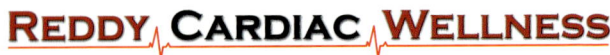

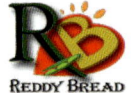

About the Author

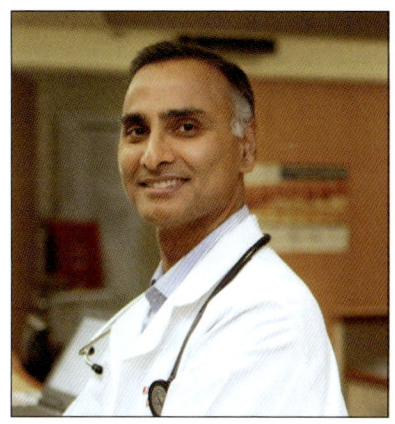

Dr. Kota J. Reddy completed his internship and performed his residency in Internal Medicine at Baylor College of Medicine. He was a research assistant in cardiology at the Stanford University in California. Dr. Reddy received his Cardiology and Interventional Fellowship at Texas Heart Institute at St. Luke's Episcopal Hospital in Houston. There he was honored to be Chief Interventional Fellow. Dr. Reddy is board certified in cardiology and is fully trained in Coronary and Peripheral Interventions. He is licensed in the state of Texas and has been in practice since 1997. Dr. Reddy's passion is the prevention and reversal of heart disease and diabetes.

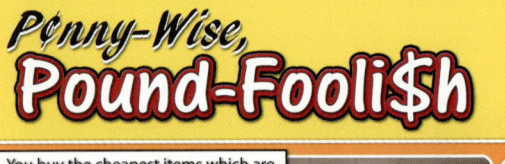

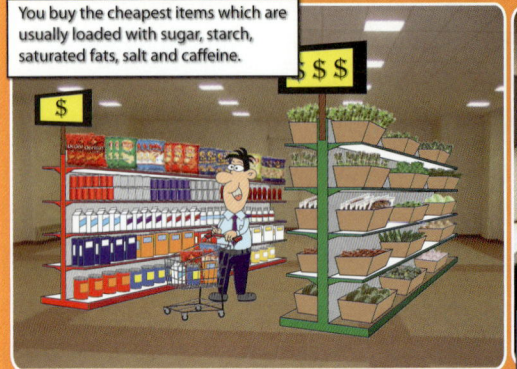

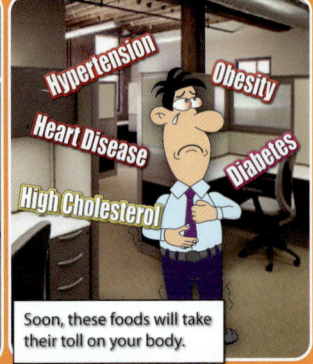

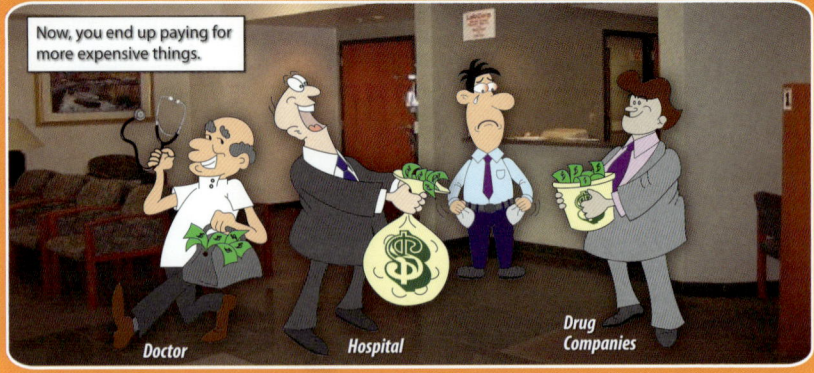

Do not complain when it's time to pay them because it's their job to take care of you when you get sick from eating junk.

For once , take the blame!

Learn to use your food as your medicine by using your grocery store as your pharmacy.

How?

By reading:
Eat this Lose that!

For more information and testimonials,
visit our website at
www.reddycardiology.com
and
www.reddybread.com

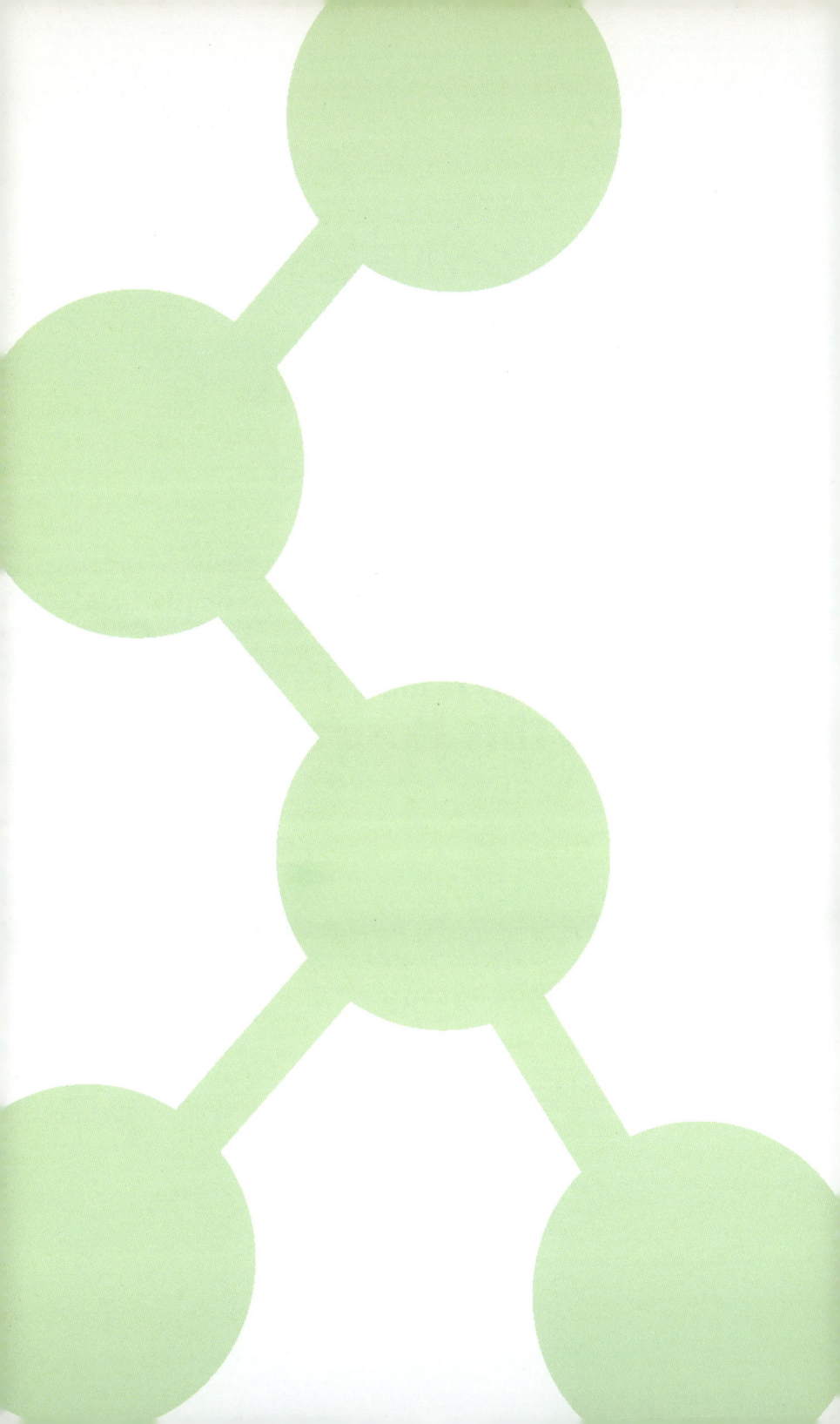